Improving your Kid's Body Image through Catholic Teaching

How Theology of the Body and Other Church Teachings Can Transform your Life

John C. Acquaviva

En Route Books and Media, LLC

Saint Louis, MO

⊕*ENROUTE*
Make the time

En Route Books and Media, LLC

5705 Rhodes Avenue

St. Louis, MO 63109

Contact us at **contact@enroutebooksandmedia.com**

Cover Credit: Sebastian Mahfood

ISBN-13: 979-8-88870-138-6

Library of Congress Control Number: 2024931775

Table of Contents

Foreword by Dr. Gregory Popcak

In his *Theology of the Body,* Pope Saint John Paul II wrote extensively about the reality of our human bodies as gifts received from God that constitute an essential part of our identity. It is through our human bodies, that is, that we may understand our purpose in life as they, in their sex, shape, size, and color, enable the connections we are able to make with other human persons and with God.

For that reason, I'm delighted to have been asked to write a short foreword for a book concerning body image, particularly as it relates to our youth who are increasingly struggling to establish their identities in a world that seems to have given up on the meaning of the human person as a rational being created in the image and likeness of God.

Now in its second edition, John Acquaviva's *Improving your Kid's Body Image through Catholic Teaching: How Theology of the Body and Other Church Teachings Can Transform your Life* provides a personable, well-reasoned explanation of the importance that body image holds within the framework of a *theology* of the body. Body image is not just about self-esteem; it's also about our capacity to love ourselves as God made us and about our capacity to love others as God made them.

- Dr. Gregory Popcak,
Founder and Executive Director,
Pastoral Solutions Institute

Preface for 2nd Edition

The Covid-19 pandemic crushed the way we see ourselves. And it didn't do any favors to the way we see others. You would think that an issue such as poor body image would take a back seat to the virus. But on the contrary, it magnified the problem. More meetings and classes via Zoom made everyone look at an image of themselves. Sometimes, all day long. Literally.

For parents, the pandemic made the problem more dismal. Take, for instance, a conversation I recently had with a parent of several teenagers with whom I shared that my wife, Alecia, and I have a big family, too, but, unlike his, ours were much younger—currently all the age of twelve and under. He laughed and said, "My friend, we both have a lot of kids, but there's a big difference: you are 'raising' kids while we are 'parenting' kids." He went on to say that with little kids Alecia and I have little problems while he has big problems. While we both have our own set of daily issues, I of course, knew what he meant. Changing diapers, scrambling to get kids to their little league games, and sleepless nights are mere nuisances compared to the barrage of complexities and difficulties that parents of older kids have to field.

All parents often feel overwhelmed by the responsibility of raising their children "right." Add in the Catholic faith and the responsibilities of parenting seem to get multiplied. While we embrace and cherish our faith, passing it on to our kids poses challenges that are unique. To be blunt, it is difficult at times to live the faith, let alone teach it to a group of young people who often find it confusing and irrelevant. But if you are reading this book, you are probably a lot like me. You see the faith as something not just worthwhile, but integral to a healthy, productive, and meaningful existence. To put it in "Catholic speak," you want your children to be the people whom God means them to be.

But every day we witness assaults on our efforts to follow God's plan within our families. Consider phones and social media for instance. Who would have guessed that things so forward-thinking and revolutionary would challenge parenting the way they do? It seems that all teenagers have smartphones, and virtually every one of them uses some form of social media. Furthermore, many adolescents have been given the same luxuries. All of this has necessitated a nightmarish level of vigilance for parents as they try to maintain a healthy balance between allowing their children the latest technology, while preventing them from diving too deeply into a world that is (or should be) reserved for adults. Too many parents have found it difficult—even *impossible*—to monitor the vastness and content of texts, Instagram, TikTok videos, and Twitter. And what about Snapchat? The instant I learned that an app was available that allowed photos to be seen for as little as *one second*, it raised a huge red flag for me and just about everyone else. Moreover, highly inappropriate subject matter garners so much attention that subtler, yet damaging images go relatively unnoticed. But even these more benign images have the potential to shatter our attempts to instill a healthy body image in our children.

Many would say that this kind of cunning subtlety is a hallmark of the Evil One. The content on smartphones and social media can be harmful; and cellphone use by our children requires constant and careful attention by those overseeing them. And it's well known that magazine, television, and internet images also invade our children's minds. To deepen the problem, those images linger and contribute to body distortion issues since our minds are made to remember. The media has been quite successful in their use of carefully crafted images to convince us that we can attain physical perfection. As a result, some of us and many of our children have become preoccupied with appearance. One of the purposes of this book is to raise awareness of, and respect for, the power of TV commercials, magazine ads, reality shows, music videos, and countless other images that have no particular category. Many of our teenagers have already taken the bait and are attempting to achieve a flawlessly beautiful face and a perfectly well-proportioned, well-toned body. Or they are increasingly anxious to an unhealthy degree because they don't have the physique they want and think they need. Some are chasing so hard after the ideal that everything else in their life has become secondary. While they might instinctively know that perfection is impossible, millions of young men and women pursue it and suffer from some form of body distortion. And more importantly, our teens start to believe that unless they are found attractive, sexy, or lean—they aren't worth much.

Results of this intense desire to "cure" a poor body image are easy to see: eating disorders, formal (often too intense) exercise regimens, cosmetic surgery, steroid use, and reckless diets. Teen body dissatisfaction is also demonstrated in a ritual known as "cutting" or other self-inflicted injuries, excessive tattoos, or self-loathing. When disproportionate amounts of time and effort are directed at self-improvement, or any type of body-destruction is practiced, daily productivity and emotional and spiritual health are compromised. And sometimes the battle starts so early in life that many spend the next several decades trying to heal the damage that began in the formative years.

And particularly troubling for parents of faith, young people who have excess anxiety over their bodies will be hampered in hearing the word of God. The anxiety and obsession will also keep them from opening their hearts to experience the power of the sacraments. If you are reading this book, you must have a sincere interest and desire to pass your Catholic faith on to your kids. And in these days filled with so many distractions, the task of parenting well and instructing children in the faith is harder than ever. When it comes to instilling in children a healthy body image and combatting the forces arrayed against it, there is little argument that it is an arduous task. Christian or not, well catechized in the faith or not, too many kids start to lose the battle of a healthy body image at a young age and never fully recover. The good news is that God stands ready to lead and empower you in the battle. I truly believe that faith is at the heart of the solution to a poor body image—in particular, the teachings of the Catholic Church.

Not every parent who reads this book will have a child who is suffering from severe body dissatisfaction, but many have a child or know of one that is affected by unhealthy concern over his or her body in some measure. Either way, we can all benefit from an improved understanding of the true meaning of the human body. This book endeavors to offer that as well as helpful parenting strategies, and I am excited to present it to you. Each chapter is inspired by a series of lectures given by Saint John Paul II entitled *Theology of the Body*, Scripture, and the teachings of the Catholic Church. Everything I have included is designed to improve understanding of the body's purpose and assist in the healing of body image issues. Understanding and valuing the church's teaching related to the body will lead to a greater appreciation of this wonderful gift. And learning how to teach and model these concepts early in your child's life may help avoid decades of tension, frustration, and even psychological trauma.

On a personal note, I teach courses in anatomy, physiology, strength and conditioning, exercise physiology, and body image— and I've never had an issue with a poor body image. Yet it makes sense that I would avidly study and develop a strong appreciation for the teachings of our former pope as they apply to the body. The theme of *Theology of the Body* elevated my awareness of the human body as a sacred gift and increased my appreciation for all that it offers.

As a college educator and advisor to young adults for almost twenty-five years, I am perhaps more aware than most that body image issues are common. Too many of my advising sessions, as well as general discussions with students, turn to concerns and anxiety about their bodies. And often these are people who seem to have little to worry about. As the instructor of a course on body image, I have had some unique conversations with students, in and out of class sessions, that have given me insight into the shame and stress that body distortion brings. At first, I responded to these anxieties just with sincere sympathy, but now I feel I have more to offer. My first book, *Improving Body Image Through Catholic Teaching*, was written to increase awareness of body image concerns and provide healing suggestions for teens and young adults. However, my focus in this book is parents. I want to empower parents to use something that they already have—their Catholic faith—to assist their children in living the healthy, meaningful life that God intends for them.

While a lot has been written on body image over the years, most of it has focused on the reasons that body dysmorphia exists. While understanding the cause is important, few have extended a level of help as meaningful and powerful as God. When I wrote that first book, I notified every friend, acquaintance, and former/current Catholic student of its availability. I received some pretty interesting, even uplifting emails from some. But nothing was more gratifying than an email from a Catholic student who took a series of classes from me a few years before. Here's what she wrote:

> This book blew me away. I read it twice in the past few days. It makes you realize how misplaced societies [*sic*] values are and how easy it is to get caught up and distracted from what's truly important.

Needless to say, I was humbled and excited to read these words as they were evidence that the book had touched someone in the way I intended. But, in reality, it wasn't *me* who inspired this young woman; it was the writers of the Catholic Catechism, and it was the words of the saints—people like Saint John Paul II and Saint Paul the Apostle. I operated as an organizer of their thoughts; I made their teaching available and welcoming, and the words, I found out, serve as a healing tool to the "average" Catholic. In this book, I make a similar effort to reach parents seeking guidance from their Catholic faith as they help their children with body image issues.

Before my introduction to JPII's *Theology of the Body*, I rarely felt that I had substantive answers for students who struggled with body distortion. Although I began teaching a course on body image years ago, the best I could do at the time for students who were struggling was listen and express sympathy. But that class did provide students a venue to open up about their struggles. In out-of-class assignments and in-class discussions (in front of strangers) they addressed their personal beliefs, struggles, and fears regarding body image. It was a start. Body image problems rarely just go away, although opening up to have discussions with a trusted friend or relative seem to help.

As I have embraced the issue of body image over the years, I've witnessed somewhat of a domino effect. Teaching a course on body image was just the first step in a series of thoughts and experiences that led to a heartfelt longing to combat this problem. The more I taught that course, the more conversations I had with young people, and the more I saw how little relief there was from the very things that trigger anxiety (e.g., magazines, television, films, images on the internet, even selfies)—the more I felt *compelled* to help.

While many experts would agree that arming yourself with good information is important, healing a poor body image requires more than learning about the history of dieting, the psychology of body distortion, and the results of a few scientific studies on eating disorders. This book limits much of that topical information and purposely omits heavy discussions on (sometimes-necessary) psychiatric help. My intent is to inspire those who battle body distortion to turn to God. Ultimately, I want to help parents help their children see the human body as gift from God and a means to gain salvation, rather than as an entity to perfect.

A comment before the conclusion of this Preface: body image issues/concerns have many synonyms. Body dissatisfaction, body dysmorphic disorder, body distortion, negative body image, and poor body image are among the most commonly used. I will use these terms interchangeably throughout this book, without intending to give one more impact than another. Also note I use the word "body" to every part of our physical being, including the face, hair, skin, eyes, hands, feet, etc.

In the book's opening chapters, there is a broad-scope discussion of the body image crisis and, using the book Genesis as the foundation, a "history" of the body and an introduction to explaining the body's purpose. The next two chapters focus on body disorder in young men and young women respectively. Both lean on the Catholic Catechism and Saint John Paul II's teachings for a solution that goes to the heart of the problem. At the center of this book (literally and figuratively) is a detailed discussion of the factors that research reveals are the chief causes of a negative body image.

The next few chapters link the problems discussed in the first section of the book to practical solutions. I directly address parents as they deal with their adolescent and teenage sons and daughters who are struggling with poor body image. The later chapters include a detailed discussion of the sacraments and the power they have to heal a poor body image. Also covered are basic myths about body image and how the words of our former pope Saint John Paul II, Holy Scripture, and the wisdom of other saints can ease the anxiety of body-related issues. But readers please take note: unless our Catholic faith—the sacraments as well as a commitment to regular prayer—is understood and embraced by parents, it will probably not transfer to our children. Parents, is your God big enough to help lift the burden of body dissatisfaction for you and the ones you love?

Introduction

Be who you are
And be that well.

— Saint Francis de Sales

One typical scalding day during the Afghanistan war, some of our soldiers on patrol suddenly got into a battle with the enemy. Sadly, within minutes many were wounded, and some died. One young private suffered severe injuries to his head. An enemy's launched grenade had done its job. Seventy surgeries later, the soldier barely recognized his own face.

Upon returning home he struggled with the thought of even going to the store, fearful of being stared at and ridiculed. In a radio interview, the soldier revealed that the only person he felt accepted him, despite his gross disfigurement, was his young bride.

Those of us who have been married for a few years understand the challenges inherent in the sacrament of marriage. But being young and married brings even greater challenges. Moreover, living life with a handicap and/or deformity adds a level of anxiety, insecurity, and complexity that most of us don't have to deal with. Then, I heard one of the more surprising revelations in the interview. It came from the soldier's wife. She admitted that she was probably more self-conscious about *her* body than he was about his. Imagine that.

Probably like most listeners that day, I was shocked by the wife's comment—but only initially. Having talked to countless young people, and having read numerous studies on body image, I wasn't surprised for very long. Still, it begs the question: What caused this woman, despite all that her husband had been through, to struggle with more body dissatisfaction issues than he did?

While the following chapters will attempt to address this, we must acknowledge that body image is an elusive and complex subject matter. It is a multidimensional minefield that involves an individual's perceptions, thoughts, and feelings about his or her body.[1] And it has been evaluated every way possible and twice on Sundays. But despite its nuanced complexity, we are closer than ever to making sense of the puzzle. There is a lot that we understand better today which can help us assist our kids in their body image struggles.

The issue of body distortion has become so widespread that it has spawned a professional journal, *Body Image*, totally dedicated to the subject. This journal was created in response to research indicating that men and women, and girls and boys, from all over the world struggle with creating a positive body image.[2] So this means it's a family issue. Sadly, I have been asked by many parents: "What could I have done better or differently?" Because body image concerns are relatively new, many parents don't realize the danger to

---

[1] J. K. Thompson, L. J. Heinberg, M. Altabe, & S. Tantleff-Dunn. (1999). *Exacting beauty: Theory, assessment, and treatment of body image disturbance.* Washington, DC.: American Psychological Association.

[2] J. Linardon. (2022, February, 25). Body Image Statistics: 47+ shocking facts and stats. https://breakbingeeating.com/body-image-statistics/

which their children are being exposed until after the damage is evident.

Regardless of who or what is to blame, the pain and frustration that parents feel for their children in these situations is universal and very real. After all, it's only natural for parents to want to protect their children from anything that harms them. We'd all like to shield our kids from the emotional scars of being bullied and of losing their first love. On a physical level, we never want to see them crack up the family car or break a leg playing soccer. And spiritually, we want to see them in church every weekend and living out their Catholic faith. We consciously and unconsciously do many things as parents to help keep them physically and mentally healthy. Keeping their body image intact is just another part of that. So, knowing the potentially harmful effects of this issue, why shouldn't we seek to know as much as possible about how to prevent it?

It will probably surprise no one to hear that the greatest incidence of body distortion is among teens and young adults. A study conducted on 45,000 Australians aged eleven to twenty-four reported that their two biggest concerns were body image and family conflict.[3] No shocker there. And believe me folks; it's everywhere we go. You can bet that similar studies conducted in the United States, Canada, or any other highly developed country would yield

---

[3] Mission Australia. (2008). National survey of young Australians 2008: key and emerging issues. Retrieved 10-12-14 from http://www.missionaustralia.com.au/document downloads/cat_view/67-youth-surveys.

the same results. And while the bitter fruit of body distortion is most commonly seen during adolescence or the teen years, the roots of the problem likely started years before.

Issues with body image are common in today's culture where we are constantly reminded of what everyone *but* God says we should value and emulate. Sometimes, it seems as though our culture—the media in particular—has declared war on our kids. It is up to us, the parents, to help our children see their bodies through God's eyes. It is God, *and God alone,* who determines the real value of our bodies. To stand by while our kids assimilate the culture's assessment of their worth is to put their emotional health and very souls in danger. Parents: our children cannot be expected to conquer severe body dissatisfaction on their own, nor should they have to.

So, what can this book offer you to aid your children in this battle? Much. As of now, there have been no aggressive efforts to address body image in relation to Scripture, the Catholic Catechism, or Saint John Paul II's *Theology of the Body.*[4] Yet, this book draws from all three. These combined sources give us a unique and powerful perspective on the meaning of the human body. They address the topic in a way that you may have not considered before, and they lead to a very different conclusion than what many children *think* the human body is for. The Catholic Church has been generous in its material on this matter and has designed its teachings for everyone, not just its faithful adults. As you read on, you

---

[4] Pope Saint John Paul II. (1997). Theology of the body: Human love in the divine plan, Pauline Press, Boston, MA. (Hereafter, citations in the text will refer to the dates of homilies, preceded by TB).

will find that the teachings are universal. This is important because the body image crisis respects no boundaries. People from every religion, gender, age, and economic status can be empowered by the church's language on this issue. Even our children can experience tremendous comfort from the church's teachings about God's purpose for the body.

In the past several years, research on body image has become ubiquitous. Most of it has been helpful in one regard or another. However, including God in the equation of developing a healthy body image is *vital*. For that reason, the primary goal of this book is to use Saint John Paul II's series of talks known as *Theology of the Body* as the guiding principle for parents as they help their children find peace with their bodies. Please note, however, that there will be no effort here to create the definitive book on the body image crisis; that has been done several times.[5] Neither is it the intention of this material to re-define or fully explain the teachings found in *Theology of the Body*, since that has been done as well.[6] While the

---

[5] Grogan, S. (2021). Body image: understanding body dissatisfaction in men, women and children, London/New York, Routledge; Bordo, S. (1993). Unbearable weight: feminism, Western culture, and the body, University of California Press, Berkeley, California; Pope, H., Phillips, K., Olivardia, R. (2000). The Adonis complex: the secret male crisis of male body obsession, The Free Press, New York.

[6] West, Christopher. (2003). Theology of the body explained: A commentary on Saint John Paul II's "Gospel of the Body", Pauline Press, Boston, MA.; Hogan, Richard. (2007). Theology of the Body in Saint John Paul II: What it means, why it matters, Word Among Us Press, Ijamsville, MD; Percy, Anthony. (2006). Theology of the body made simple, Pauline Press, Boston, MA.

former Pope's revolutionary teachings in those lectures are the primary inspiration for this book, you will see only a modest number of direct quotes scattered throughout. But keep in mind that Saint John Paul II linked his *Theology of the Body* work directly to Scripture and the Catholic Catechism—both of which are heavily relied upon here. Still, this book is not for theologians; it is for people like you and me (being a parent of four) who seek to raise happy, healthy, and holy children.

Despite the limited direct references to *Theology of the Body*, it may be helpful to provide a little background on it. While these writings have recently gained popularity in some Catholic circles, they haven't always been adequately understood. And not all of *Theology of the Body* is relevant to raising children. Therefore, this book is written expressly to bring the basic concepts of these marvelous teachings to parents in a manner that makes them easy to apply to everyday life—especially where body image and young people are concerned.

The *Theology of the Body* teachings can be purchased in book form and several authors have made valiant attempts to explain the contents for lay people. But despite the complexity of these writings, the central message from Saint John Paul II can be stated simply: God created the body as a "sign" of His own divine mystery. This is why the former pope speaks of the body as both a theology (a way to come to know God) *and* as a language (a tool to reveal ourselves to others). Further, in his Son, "God has revealed his innermost secret: God himself is an eternal exchange of love, Father, Son, and Holy Spirit, and he has destined us to share in that exchange."[7] That is, an *appropriate* use of the body—in relationship with himself and others—is at the core of God's divine plan, and that is why children need guidance from a young age on defining and discerning what is appropriate. While a full comprehension of this message may be difficult for most young people to grasp, this book will help parents to explain it to their children in age-appropriate ways.

It seems that we often fail to see the greatness of our bodies; we take them for granted. While we marvel at God's creations—snow-peaked mountains, cascading streams, strutting peacocks, and so on—nothing shouts more loudly of his greatness than does the intricacy of the human being.

Children, easily distracted and consumed by so many poisonous images, are most susceptible to a basic lack of appreciation for the marvel that is their body. It is vital that parents help them see the human person as the greatest revelation of God's existence. Every child since Adam and Eve has been created in God's image. It is through their bodies that they demonstrate God's reality and express what is in their soul. To children, this concept can be more baffling than a class on genetics. It can lead to good questions such as, "How can we reflect God even though our bodies are not perfect?" and, "How can our Catholic faith make a difference in the way I see my body?"

Without solid answers to questions like these, our tendency is to allow others to interpret the worth of our children's bodies. Indeed, in an environment saturated with stimuli and lacking God's

---

[7] *Catechism of the Catholic Church*, No. 221.

word, any person could fall prey to a misunderstanding of the worth of the body. And children are especially vulnerable. I have written this book because I firmly believe that God must be at the center of a healthy body image. I want you to convince you, too, and help you pass that truth on to your children.

In fact, one of the primary objectives of this book is to educate parents. They are the ones on the front lines of the battle for the minds of their children. Parents are the ones tasked with helping their children understand God's plan for their bodies while negating the barrage of media messages that constantly lay siege. And please, never underestimate the number of distractions to lead us astray from the true meaning of the body. But I bring good news: the truth lies within our Catholic faith. The church's teaching can help us know God better, develop our understanding of why He made us, and help us and our children live out the implications in today's world.

The Catholic faith is not designed to erase all the challenges of our children's lives, but to inform, encourage, and strengthen them to overcome those challenges when they occur. Recall the opening story: a soldier's body was distorted from a roadside bomb—and thus began a life-long challenge. You held your children in your arms from the first few moments of life—and thus began another life-long challenge. A Catholic parent's role is to take what the church offers, embrace it, and pass it on to our kids. Although our children may face tough times on the road to a healthy body image, there is *more* good news: God is able and always available to help us impact how our children see themselves.

Chapter 1

It Started in the Garden

Love tends upward to God and is not occupied with the things of earth. Love also will be free from all worldly affections, so that its inner vision does not become dimmed, nor does it let itself be trapped by any temporal interest or downcast by misfortune.

—Thomas à Kempis, *The Imitation of Christ*

It's Friday, you're running behind, Kid #2 still needs to be picked up from his Scout meeting, the traffic's thickening and, *of course*, the person in front of you at the checkout has enough items to fill a small warehouse. You just stopped in for a few items for an already-late dinner, and now you find yourself staring at what we all stare at when we're stuck in line.

Those dreaded glossy magazine covers—yet that capture your attention.

You know the ones: "24/7 Hot Looks!" or, "Get a Beach Body in *ONLY* 8 Days" and the old standby, "Get Your Flat Belly Back with these 3 easy Steps!"

Just as the toys, gum, and candy are purposely placed at a four-year-old's eye level, these magazines are not placed at our eye level by chance. And they are very effective at doing two things: they play on our desire to know details or gossip about celebrities, and they play on our fears—particularly the fear in how we view our own bodies. These magazine covers are clever, even cunning. The number of blurbs seems limitless, and they are always in the foreground of an image of a beautiful young woman with very few clothes on. Think about how such images and words play on *your* body image. As parents, we've (thankfully) conquered teenage anxiety and we're (probably) over the near-obsession with beauty and sexiness. But before the celery and organic milk are on the counter, your gum-snapping teenage daughter is already on page thirty-seven, reading tips on how to reduce her already alarmingly trim waistline.

And the magazine covers are just one of many outlets that play on our deeply-rooted fears. Television commercials, social media sites, airbrushed magazine pics, imaginative internet ads, and even emails sent to personal accounts are all designed to relentlessly pursue unsuspecting victims. We actually start to believe that sweat-gushing workouts, constantly slathering on makeup, or hunting for the latest fashions will lead us to happiness and contentment. This is not to say that exercise and personal hygiene don't play a proper role in our self-worth and emotional well-being. A certain level of fear in, say, gaining weight is actually healthy. But aspiring to a specific look—which is often confined to a particular age, skin color, and body type—can be self-defeating and dangerous.

The disturbingly popular TV reality shows—*The Bachelor* and *The Bachelorette* and ones like it—are prime examples of the fang-toothed predators that swim in our collective waters. For those somehow unfamiliar with these shows, their premise is that one single young person (the bachelor or bachelorette) is courted by dozens of suitors. The one being courted gradually narrows the field until only one young person remains, supposedly to be their mate or (perhaps) spouse. The wizards-in-charge (the writers and producers) are adept at making even the most alluring people on the planet feel inadequate. One need only see the commercials for these shows to know that both the suitors and the one being pursued are young, beautiful, and in-shape—without exception. But these shows do illustrate a dirty truth: even if you're all the above, you may still end up alone if you're not pursued by someone of equal or greater attributes.

It's a given that many watch such shows solely as entertainment, dismissing any spiritual or emotional distress that they may bring. But we need to respect how shows like this play on our basic fears and insecurities as well as our faith life.

Character traits such as humility and modesty seem to be non-existent in these and similar TV shows. But we know that pride or self-love—those thoughts and/or acts meant to serve ourselves—stifle our attempt to find our true purpose and participate in self-giving love. As Scripture tells us, "True love does not contain fear, in fact perfect love denies fear" (1 John 4:18). What's sad is that fear seems to be the underlying emotion driving such reality shows. Consider the aforementioned fear of being alone. Many young people are frazzled at the very thought of being alone, so "competitions" like *The Bachelorette* can stir up a beehive of suppressed feelings. It is all-too-easy to let TV shows and such dictate our feelings rather than allow God to guide them. Whether or not we, as parents, allow our children to watch these shows is not the only problem. Remember the smartphone you gave them for Christmas? That'll sure challenge any kid to be virtuous. And you're not always at home, either. If they're not watching *The Bachelor*, they're probably watching other shows that can have a similar impact on their impressionable minds.

So, if fear leads us to react or think in a fashion contrary to our Creator's desire for us, what should our attitude be? For the answer, let's look at God's plan for us from the beginning of time, when the human race was new and fresh. The Genesis story is full of powerful religious truths that communicate God's intention for us.

God created man with two components: the spiritual and the physical. Both components were involved in the fall of man into sin. Eve was the first to fall spiritually by listening to and being tricked by the serpent. But to fall spiritually, her body had to cooperate. Eve's body followed where her mind and soul wanted to go. Saint John Paul II says that Eve, although fallen, could have been restored at this point since Adam remained intact as her sinless partner. But tragically, Adam also buckled to temptation and these acts of sin continue to bear bitter fruit. When called by God, Adam answered, "I heard you in the garden; but I was afraid, because I was naked, so I hid myself" (Gen 3:10). It is in the Garden of Eden that man and woman were ashamed of their bodies for the first time.[1]

---

[1] 2/20/80 TB.

Before the fall, God declared that he liked what he had made. He saw his creation, man, said it was not just good but *very good*. Man was indeed the pinnacle of his creative work. The human person was to govern over all of God's other creations. More importantly, he and she were created to reflect God in the world (Gen 1:26). As the Catholic Catechism tells us:

> The human body shares in the dignity of "the image of God": it is a human body precisely because it is animated by a spiritual soul, and it is the whole human person that is intended to become, in the body of Christ, a temple of the Spirit: Man, though made of body and soul, is a unity. Through his very bodily condition he sums up in himself the elements of the material world. Through him they are thus brought to their highest perfection and can raise their voice in praise freely given to the Creator. For this reason, man may not despise his bodily life. Rather he is obliged to regard his body as good and to hold it in honor since God has created it and will raise it up on the last day.[2]

God created us to reflect the love he has for us, and to share that love with others. Now, for your teenagers, this should not read as a *carte blanche* to sleep around. When we look at our bodies and those of others, we should see God and His mystery—and *only* God and his mystery. Alas, the bitter fruit of sin was pride, selfishness, and lust. And these skewed heart inclinations gave birth to the

---

[2] *Catechism of the Catholic Church*, No. 274.

thought that we could live independently of God's intention that we love and respect our bodies as a gift from him. To any parent of a teenager, communicating this notion can sound as scary as scaling a cliff without a carabiner. Nevertheless, it is our responsibility to do battle for our children's hearts and minds. And we can persevere if we arm ourselves with select quotes from Scripture, the catechism, and *Theology of the Body* (for specifics, see chapter nine).

Saint John Paul II says that our physical being alone gives evidence of the existence of God, or what the pope calls the "God Question."[3] God desires a relationship and gives us the freedom to offer our bodies as well as our hearts to him. This is the essence of *Theology of the Body*: the body is the true "sign" that God exists. It makes "seen" what was until the creation of our bodies, "unseen." That is, God being pure invisible spirit intended his love for us to be visible, so he created the human body in his image (Gen 1:27). Further, the pope tells us that the use of our body for love of others is the way we reflect the relationship in the Trinity. This is the appropriate use of the body—the use that glorifies God.[4]

We can model this for our children and encourage them to see the beauty of the body through work, play, and in service to one another. Moreover, by frequently calling attention to the fact that work, play, and service are at the core of God's intention for the body, parents can reframe their child's entire view of the body. But this doesn't happen by saying it only once—it has to be affirmed often starting when they're just out of diapers.

---

[3] Catholic Church and Saint John Paul II (1995). *Crossing the Threshold of Hope.* New York, NY: Random House.

[4] 1/13/82 TB

Through the language of the body as a gift that can serve God, the pope seeks to answer two vital questions: (1) What does it mean to be human? and, (2) How do I live a life in a way that brings true happiness and fulfillment? Saint John Paul II says "The body, and it alone, is capable of making visible what is invisible, the spiritual and divine. [The body] was created to transfer into the visible reality, the invisible mystery hidden in God from time immemorial, and thus to be a sign of it. [The body] is the fundamental fact of human existence."[5] So it is our physical bodies that clarify the mystery of existence.

One of the main reasons that these words seem counterintuitive is that so many people, even some theologians (primarily in the past), have de-emphasized the physical body and packed all worth into the soul. *Theology of the Body* does not downplay the soul in any way but raises the importance of the body. Children who are taught the value of their soul as it is expressed in a respect for their body as God's gift will have a much healthier and holier outlook on their lives.

However, salacious advertisements, immodest fashion, television shows, and countless other graphic images have distorted the meaning of the body as a gift. The body has become so objectified that sometimes before the age of ten our understanding of it is skewed. We defer to what *society* dictates for our bodies, not what *God* wants. Far from being acknowledged as a gift, the body is of-

---

[5] 2/20/80 TB.

ten portrayed as means to an end.[6] It is used to sell a product, to "sell" oneself, and sometimes both.

For example, consider cheerleaders for professional sports teams. The common reasoning is that their presence and activity improve team spirit. Okay. And the women themselves would probably say that accepting such a job is simply a way to support their favorite team. Oh, and that it pays well. The truth, whether it's admitted or not, is that they are being used *and* doing the using. By taking the job, the cheerleader enters the arena of body distortion. Let's face it—they are being used for their bodies. Period. Yet at the same time, they and their employers are responsible for contributing to society's distorted views on appropriate uses of the body. Or as my wife says just about every time NFL cheerleaders are shown bouncing on-screen, "What does *that* have to do with football?" Here's a question worth exploring indeed.

Dressing in such ways will certainly attract and help sustain male viewership (arguably the reason cheerleaders are hired) even as they use their role to enhance their self-worth or improve their financial standing (reasons for seeking such employment). And to complicate the matter further, the average male viewer is (knowingly or not) encouraged to desire that his girlfriend or wife look like the cheerleader. Meanwhile, the average female viewer internalizes (knowingly or not) the message that her worth is based upon her ability to attain to that level of beauty or sexiness. Therefore, both creating and accepting this job has consequences for society, and everyone involved is culpable to some degree.

---

[6] 1/9/80 TB.

It should be noted that without the "cheerleader effect" in place, the beauty/fashion industry, most magazines, pornography, etc., would fail as businesses. They all endure by promoting and relying upon competitiveness among young women. Fat bank accounts are the result of women demanding to look not only *their* best, but better than all other women. And it's not just women pressuring themselves. Males can apply undue pressure on females to maintain that a certain look, or they can encourage the illusion that physical perfection is possible. Lately, this deception has been successfully marketed to a male audience as well—they call the resulting male persona "metro-sexual."

In either case, the justification is sinister, and it further deepens the distortion of the body's purpose. Just as Adam and Eve first saw each other as pure love, our youth are called to see the body as a gift designed to express authentic love.[7] In fact, conflicting or opposing views of this divine love are what provide the basis for a society filled with poor self-worth and negative body images. The madness and distortion have born bitter fruit—many of our young people have bought into the lie that they have dignity only if they attain physical beauty or can effectively arouse and attract others.

Research has been clear in demonstrating that the more we are exposed to images of "perfect" bodies the more we turn our thoughts, intentions, and energy toward making ourselves perfect. This is known as the Social Comparison Theory. When our children aggressively seek to build a flawless body, it puts them on a

---

[7] 5/30/84 TB.

dangerous road for two fundamental reasons. First, they may become self-centered, and thus, selfish.

When something takes an inordinate amount of time and effort to perfect, all other aspects of life will fade like a melting glacier. Specifically, a greedy pursuit of perfection will result in diminished pursuit of God and what he has called us to do: serve him by caring for and loving one another. Ignoring the call of God assumes many faces. It results in having very little (or no) time to be a caring friend, teammate, sibling, or son/daughter. Few inclinations are more effective at hauling us away from God than a desire to spend countless hours and emotional energy striving for the perfect body. We can actually begin to believe that with enough time and effort it is possible to *be* perfect! Lack of insight and experience make young people especially susceptible to this kind of false thinking.

Second, they may think that God is not a basic necessity. Thinking that they don't need God may seem a normal thought for adolescents, teenagers, and many young adults, but it is deadly. It puts their very salvation in jeopardy. It is vital to our spiritual well-being that we respect the powerful lure of a desire for perfection and acknowledge the role that God plays in helping us to defeat it, and further that he is the one who gives meaning and purpose to life.

But parents, it must also be said that when *we* fail to seek out God our kids can assume that they don't need him either. So, this is a great example of where our actions and words probably contribute greatly to the outcome of our child's overall health.

Both reasons directly deal with understanding and embracing the call to love God and show that love through our actions toward one another, all of which can override prideful desires. The love that Scripture calls us to redirects our time and efforts to serving and meeting the needs of others. This is important because knowing and accepting our proper vocation leads to a life of unselfishness and true fulfillment. Introducing these basic principles of Christian living to children at a young age will enable them to grow in understanding that the human body is God's greatest gift. So read here: Use this body only in case of emergency, friendships, service to others, at play, employment, and marriage!

It is Saint Paul who pleads with us to offer our bodies to God, to make them a living sacrifice, to make our experiences actual acts of worship (Rom 12:1). Without the physical body, we wouldn't have the means to concretely show love. The physical acts of love not only bond us to one another, but they bond us to God and unfold for us the full understanding of life's purpose. Reflect on what Saint John Paul II said about our vocation:

Each one of you too is confronted by the challenge of giving full meaning to your life, the one life you are given to live. You are young and you want to live. But you must live fully and with a purpose. You must live for God; you must live for others. And no one can live this life for you. The future is yours, but the future is above all a call and a challenge to "keep" your life by giving it up, by "losing" it-as the Gospel has reminded us-by sharing it through loving service of others. You are called to be witnesses of the paradox that Christ proposes. "He who loves his life loses it, he who hates his life in this world will keep it for eternal life" (John 12:25). And the measure of ready to love, is to assist, to help-in the family, at work, at recreation-those who are near and those who are far away. Also your success will be the measure of your generosity. You, too, be courageous! The world needs convinced and fearless witnesses. It is not enough to discuss; it is necessary to act! . . . live in grace, abide in His love, putting into practice the whole moral law, nourishing your soul with the Body of Christ, taking advantage of the Sacrament of Penance periodically and seriously. Always consider, with seriousness and generosity, whether the Lord might not also be calling some of you.[8]

While this is surely a beautiful insight from our former pope, it's not something that your teens are likely to be reading in their down time. So, I encourage you to have a discussion or two with your children about vocation. This talk can be friendly, basic, and have two general points. First, introduce the term "vocation" and explain what it means regarding their existence. Using some of the words from the above quote from Saint John Paul II would be a good place to start. Terms like "purpose/meaning" and "live for God" can give shape and direction to your talk. But make no mistake—this can be a tough conversation to have. And it may initially fall on deaf ears since all seeds don't land on fertile ground (Matt 13:8).

The second purpose of a talk on vocation is to develop your child's understanding that what he or she does contribute to socie-

---

[8] Catholic Church and Saint John Paul II (1997). *The Meaning of Vocation*, Strongsville, OH: Scepter Publishers.

ty in a meaningful way—whether working at the local fast food joint as a teen or becoming a surgeon. Most people, Catholics included, tend to associate the term "vocation" with becoming a priest or a nun, teaching, or doing some type of mission work. The fact is that a vocation involves saying "yes" to the state of life God is specifically calling you to—be it religious life, married life, or the single life. Our vocation or "calling" in life is the path that will allow us to serve God best. It will aid us in becoming the person he created us to be; it will lead to our increasing holiness when lived sincerely and well.

It is important to distinguish between a job and a vocation. We can hold many jobs throughout our lives, yet most of us are called to just one specific vocation. A job is generally something we go to every day; it takes up much of the day and pays some of the bills. If we fail to see how our days contribute to improving society, then we should reconsider our job or our motives for doing it. A vocation should bring a sense of fulfillment to our lives while also fulfilling our God-given purpose. Ideally, we can help our children to find a path in life that affirms their vocation and provides a fulfilling job path as well.

We can help teach our kids that vocations cannot be fulfilled without the body, providing yet another opportunity for youth to view the body through the eyes of God. As an extension of this, we can also regularly remind our children of the other wonders of the body. All of this plays a role in the universal vocation of glorifying God. The good news is that those reminders can come at times that are natural and conversational—during grace at dinner, driving home from band or sports practice, and while doing crafts. And if you feel really bold, you can throw in some of the most meaningful ways to use the body such as the display of affection and gratitude towards one another (embracing, kissing, etc.), and honoring God (kneeling, genuflecting, or singing a hymn at Mass). Whether your child fully realizes or appreciates it, every action or activity that we engage in is an authentic gift and should be understood and appreciated in that way. When a society becomes consumed with the immoral and unethical roles of the body (common and regular temptations), it becomes easy for us to forget the beautiful simplicity in which the body is used in very noble, dignified, and holy ways.

And remember, don't let the media or anything else determine your worth. Let God do that.

Chapter 2

Why the Madness

Brothers and sisters:
You are not in the flesh;
on the contrary, you are in the spirit,
if only the Spirit of God dwells in you.
Whoever does not have the Spirit of Christ does not belong to him.
If the Spirit of the one who raised Jesus from the dead dwells in you,
the one who raised Christ from the dead
will give life to your mortal bodies also,
through his Spirit that dwells in you.

—Romans 8: 9, 11-13

In the midst of writing this book, I heard a remarkable comment: One of my colleagues told me that his college-age son didn't think that famous swimsuit model Kate Upton was good-looking. Instead, brace yourself; he said she was too fat. My immediate thought was: "This is where we've come regarding body image and body size? A typical guy is calling a woman who is five feet ten inches tall, who weighs 137 pounds and whose dress size is eight, fat?" My next thought was: "I am going to put that in my book!" In fact, how could I *not* put that in this book? The young man probably didn't give his remark a second thought, let alone imagine that it would end up on these humble pages. But it *did* end up in this book and deservedly so. It's a sad commentary on how we see each other and ourselves. Kate Upton is fat? Really? Now if you don't know who Kate Upton is, Google an image or two of her, shake your head in astonishment that someone labeled her fat, and read on.

Guest speakers are an integral part of the body image class I teach to college students. I've invited everyone from a plastic surgeon to an editor of a women's magazine to share their work experiences. When I first taught the class several years ago, I asked the editor to speak to my class. I asked her to focus on the way she manipulates her photos. She admitted to always changing *something* on the model (e.g., smoothing wrinkles, erasing age spots, etc.) or something else in the photo (e.g., deleting unnecessary background objects). In addition to her personal experiences, her presentation included a discussion about other popular magazines and how their images were typically enhanced using Adobe Photoshop, something that was novel at the time. For this particular semester, the class was mostly female.

Now, as a professor of twenty years tenure, I've seen it all: rolling eyes, texting, dozing, and the heavy sighs indicating sheer boredom. But the students in this class were *glued* to the editor. They hung on her every word as if she were Moses speaking from the mountaintop. And when she completed her presentation, there was an uncomfortable silence in the air. Then a modest-looking girl seated near the back of the room spoke up. Looked around the room with tears in her eyes she asked, "Why do they do that to us?" It was an unforgettable moment. Her words were more than a question—they were a potent statement. Her comment peeled back the layers of delusion in the body image crisis. It revealed the despondency, frustration, and life-long drama of this issue.

College professors (like yours truly), sociologists, and a variety of researchers have identified many of the factors that lead to a poor body image, although none are absolute. Some causes are so powerful they've challenged men and women who have an otherwise healthy view of their bodies.[1] On an individual basis, it is difficult to determine which factor will have the most impact. Still, a great deal of research has been completed on this topic, and it's worth the time and space to devote an entire chapter to what we've learned. So, let's take a more in-depth look at some of the contributors to a poor body image.

Magazines

Despite being created in 1988 as a multi-use graphics editor, Adobe Photoshop remains a household name due to its ability to manipulate photographs in a variety of ways and continues to be used heavily to this day. I recall seeing a TV commercial about a mom who was looking through a stack of family photos. She was annoyed that none of the photos captured all her young children smiling at the same time. So, she implanted the face of one of her sons on another photo and, *voilà*, created the perfect family pic-

---

[1] Grogan, S. (2021). Body image: understanding body dissatisfaction in men, women and children, London/New York, Routledge; Bordo, S. (1993). Unbearable weight: feminism, Western Culture, and the body, University of California Press, Berkeley, California.

ture. Now, if the everyday person can do this to create a perfect and lasting image, think what a clever and experienced editor could do with the pictures of models and actors. Although the perfect person does not exist, basic computer software has created the illusion that it's possible.

Women's fashion magazine covers and the photos within are notorious for featuring beautiful women with striking eyes, revealing clothing, and perfect teeth and smiles. These images are common, and it's impossible *not* to be drawn to them. And fitness magazine models seem to be identical to their fashion model counterparts in age and beauty, but with slightly more muscle tone. Their attire is different (even jock-like), yet equally revealing.

Magazines designed for male readership use a similar in tactic to attract attention. They feature uber-fit males who are youthful, handsome, and have better physical attributes than anyone we know. But these are not the Charles Atlas types of your father's generation. These men are trimmed and tweaked Adonis-like statuettes with increased muscle structure and low body fat, sometimes both of which are extreme. No matter the reason for this change, males (and certainly boys) have taken notice, and the result is that a greater percentage of them feel inadequate about their bodies. Hollywood actors add to this equation. Good examples are The Rock, Chris Hemsworth, Zac Efron, and the multitudes who play a superhero – man or woman.

<u>Why magazines matter</u>: I once read that it takes days to perfect lighting, shadows, and angles to capture that playful, "impromptu" moment. Magazines are selling us on the idea that the woman with the sparkling eyes in the image is carefree and whimsical. We be-

come convinced that she is without worry or concern, and it becomes difficult *not* to want to be that person. She is the center of attention, alluring, sexy—she seems to have it all. Regardless of the product being sold, our senses are being invaded and our desire to be that model is amplified.

While Adobe Photoshop was originally designed and priced for major fashion magazine editors, it wasn't long before editors of every type of magazine learned how to quickly remove age spots, lessen wrinkles, whiten teeth, thicken hair, and (what I was told to be the most popular use) remove veins from the white of the eye. Just glance at any photo, especially a close-up, and you'll rarely see any redness in the model's eyes.

To no one's surprise, it has been realized that readers/viewers (women being the most impacted) make instant comparisons to the models as they look. The comparisons linger for hours following the time spent viewing these images.[2] Just one glance at the cover is enough to trigger feelings of inadequacy. Imagine the impact a weekly or monthly subscription might have.

It's normal, at least on occasion, to compare ourselves to others. However, two issues arise when we try to regularly "measure up." First, we compare ourselves to an incredibly high standard. Models who are selected to advertise eye-care products have un-

---

[2] Major, B., Testa, M., & Bylsma, W.H. (1991). Responses to upward and downward social comparisons: The impact of esteem-relevance and perceived control. In Suls, J. & Wills, T. (Eds.), *Social comparison: Contemporary theory and research* (pp. 237-260). Hillsdale, NJ: Lawrence Erlbaum,1991.

commonly stunning eyes, and those who appear in hair product ads have unnaturally thick and silky hair. In addition, those who model fitness attire are clearly blessed with the rare combination of a high metabolic rate and/or the discipline to exercise daily. Frankly, it's a game that should not be played. Talk about the high risk of losing. Second, the fact that these exemplary physical features are further refined with the power of Adobe Photoshop means no reader could possibly meet the standard created. Yet, many of us try. It is in the attempt to meet the perfect standard that frustration increases, and anxiety sets in. It's no accident that magazines head the list in this chapter. What's viewed as normal (your teen plastering pages out of those magazines all over her bathroom mirror and bedroom door) should be seen as harmful. While she wants to emulate those images, the reality is that such photos cause more angst than motivation.

There is no mystery to the purpose of these magazine photos. They are meant to convince the reader that his or her life will be similar to the lives being portrayed in the photo (happy, rewarding, etc.). All we must do is buy the product they advertise.

Take, for instance, this "Jedi Mind Trick": When the cover girl is the focus, the male in the picture is often looking at her with lust or affection. The same goes for many men's magazines where the women in the pictures appear to be in awe of the chiseled male models. In both cases, feelings of insecurity are sure to envelop the reader. People looking at these models will not only see the perfect body and face but will be led to suppose that having the perfect body and face will necessarily bring joy, affection, respect, and love. Thus, we are more inclined to purchase the product advertised.

Worse still, we buy the lie that attaining bodily perfection will lead to true contentment.

Note that phone apps called Magic Eraser and Object Eraser now exist, but these two apps appear to address "photobombing" and other distractions in a photo, rather than putting an emphasis on improving skin tone and removing wrinkles. But other phone apps like TouchRetouch more directly address facial and body imperfections which allows the average smartphone user to use similar tools as the editor of a fashion magazine who uses Photoshop.

<u>Magazines and parenting</u>: Magazines like the ones described pose challenges for parents. But like most points made in this chapter, the way to deal with this problem is probably obvious. In the case of magazines, simply don't buy them. And if they do slip inside the cracks of your home, don't let them collect dust on your coffee table. We have enough reminders of how "imperfect" we are. Even the occasional purchase of such magazines can give your kids the idea that you aspire to be like the models in the photos or that it's okay if they do. And don't let your kids buy them either. To keep your kids away from these magazines entirely is not realistic twenty-first century thinking, but minimizing their exposure to them will help. It might eliminate a probable cause of body image problems, as well as allow you to make a statement about their unhealthy potential. Further, be sure to discuss early on (in adolescence) Adobe Photoshop software and its effect. In particular, use one or more of these magazines to point out specific ways that it is used (e.g., the models have no wrinkles even when smiling, no veins in their eyes, and no pores in their skin). You can also watch

YouTube videos together to see a professional use Adobe Photoshop software to make (sometimes extreme) alterations to photos of models or ordinary people (see https://youtu.be/YP31r70_QNM and https://youtu.be/6TFbWA5wV78).

As just a point of interest, while I was viewing images of Kate Upton, I found several normal-looking and even unflattering photos of her. You see, without a team of experts, the perfect lighting and setting, Adobe Photoshop, and a professional photographer, even *she* can look normal. Well, close to normal.

Television and the Internet

We all know most of our youth devote a lot of time to television watching and internet use. To simplify things, researchers tend to condense watching television, using the internet, and playing video games into "screen time," which has exploded to nine hours per day for teens-pre and post pandemic.[3] We can safely assume that the commercials, music videos, streamed movies, reality shows, internet images, and videos play a role in the increase of body-related anxieties among our young people. Further, many

---

[3] Nagata, J. M., Cortez, C. A., Cattle, C. J., Ganson, K. T., Iyer, P., Bibbins-Domingo, K., & Baker, F. C. (2022). Screen time use among US adolescents during the COVID-19 pandemic: findings from the Adolescent Brain Cognitive Development (ABCD) study. *JAMA Pediatrics, 176*(1), 94-96; Common Sense Medai. (2015, November 3). Landmark Report: U.S. Teens Use an Average of Nine Hours of Media Per Day, Tweens Use Six Hours. https://www.commonsensemedia.org/press-releases/landmark-report-us-teens-use-an-average-of-nine-hours-of-media-per-day-tweens-use-six-hours

movies and streamed shows target a vulnerable young audience at a time in life when issues about their body image are just developing.

Why television and the internet matter: The formula for much of the programming is a perfect petri dish for developing a poor body image. We talked in the first chapter about Reality TV and all its backstabbing, competitive, bikini-clad undertones. The internet, with its R- and X-rated content is so easily accessed and problematic that it could be another chapter by itself. All this funnels into the same problem: youth exposed to these images will eventually compare themselves to those on screen—contestants and actors who have been hand-selected for their youth and attractiveness levels. Again, it is a contest no one can win. The constant comparisons eventually deliver a crushing blow to their body image.

Television watching/streaming, internet usage, and parenting: I'd like to offer a caution for parents who tell themselves that watching reality TV and browsing the internet is for entertainment purposes only. The next time you're preparing family dinner while such things play in the background, lend an ear to what's happening on that screen. It is established fact that TV shows, videos, and photos leave long-lasting images that play a role in creating a distorted self-view. To demonstrate the power of TV on body image, researchers condensed the results of twenty-five experimental studies. They found that the body image of participants was more negatively affected after viewing thin models compared to viewing average to plus-sized models, or inanimate objects.[4] Think of it as *Baywatch* versus *The Biggest Loser*. It's not hard to consider the impact that these images and words can have in a month, a year, and even decades of TV and internet viewing. One last suggestion: consider website blockers. Some of the better ones are even free.

Social Media

In reality, social media is an extension of television, movies, and magazines. However, it literally puts images in the hands of the user and does so at lightning speed. Leaving the addictive component for another conversation, social media should be acknowledged as the quickest rising factor in this discussion. As with the other factors, teens and young adults rarely realize the harmful impact. They are more apt to see their participation in social media simply as a means of networking or keeping up with "friends." Those who have access to or are "followers" of Instagram, Facebook, and Twitter view so many images in such fleeting time that it poses a unique and formidable challenge for researchers to capture the true impact.

Still, it has taken no time at all for health professionals to investigate social media's impact on body image. Not surprisingly, they have shown that a barrage of provocative and appealing photos and videos—mainly from Twitter, Facebook, Instagram, and TikTok—

---

[4] Groesz, L., Levine, M., & Murnen, S. (2002). The effect of experimental presentation of thin media images on body satisfaction: a meta-analytic review. *International Journal of Eating Disorders, 31,* 1-16.

damage the body image health of the viewer.[5] Like fashion magazine editors, some site-owners carefully select and manipulate photos (unintentionally) causing the viewers to feel inadequate. In fact,
the pure volume of images on these sites is bound to cause some
issues. The poses, attire, and effort put into creating the image of a
perfect life create a particular challenge for the parent. How do you
allow your teens some freedom but protect them against some of
the dangers that freedom causes? Hold that thought.

Why social media matters: The popularity of social media has
been well established. Statistics show that nearly seventy-five percent of teens are known to be regular users. The chances your kid is
not part of this number is unlikely. The combination of viewing
images and reading/hearing comments from others about the attractiveness of those images (sometimes, those they consider to be
true friends) makes a powerful contribution to the world of negative body image. In her book *American Girls: Social Media and the
Secret Lives of Teenagers* (2016), Nancy Jo Sales says, "For many
girls, the pressure to be considered 'hot' is felt on a nearly continual
basis online." Few things take away a young person's chances to be
virtuous than the extraordinary efforts to be thought of as "hot."
Studying the effects of social media is complicated by the fact that
it changes at such a rapid rate. This makes it hard for even researchers to study the problem for extended periods (an important

---

[5] Franchina, V., & Coco, G. L. (2018). The influence of social media
use on body image concerns. *International Journal of Psychoanalysis and
Education, 10*(1), 5-14.

benefit in the realm of research). And by the way, who would have conceived some of these social media platforms just a decade ago?

Incidentally, a recent Google search for "How does Snapchat work?" retrieved an explanation that began with, "Despite the obvious naughty uses . . ." Wait—they just used the word "naughty" and yet some parents dismiss it as a cute app?

Many current social media outlets allow, even promote side-stepping modesty for teens. With Snapchat alone, modesty seems to have little chance. And who knows what technology lies around the corner? What kind of challenges will it pose for parents as well as children who are battling a poor body image?

<u>Social media and parenting</u>: While teenagers have felt misunderstood by their parents for centuries, it seems that social media has singlehandedly widened that gap in a snap. And you can be sure that teens are clever at making their parents *feel* that they are in the loop of their social media actions when they are not. Dismissing the impact of social media on your child's body image would be analogous to seeing reality TV as mere entertainment. To be truthful, I wish I didn't feel the need to continually press in on the role that constant and appealing images have on young minds. I imagine you already feel somewhat overwhelmed, and this book is only in its early chapters. But I want to encourage you to hang in there. Read the entire book, and then let's plan to address all the culprits—social media issues included.

Video Platforms

I was recently watching an hour-long news program in which the host would bring each guest on for a video interview. Any viewer would note that many of the guests regularly became distracted by themselves. That is, they would check themselves out the same way we all pass by a series of mirrors, just fleeting glimpses, but a lot of them. Every user of Zoom, the most popular video platform, knows that each participant sees a business card-size image of all attendees of the meeting. With that comes the almost impossible task of *not* looking at yourself, at least periodically.

Why video platforms matter: With the onset of the pandemic, a major form of communication such as any type of meeting – especially for work, as well as for K-college classes, Zoom (or other platforms) became necessary. As a result, body image issues are running higher than ever. The reason for this is probably obvious since so many use this platform. Me included. What that means is that we've spent hours looking directly not only at other people, but also, of course, ourselves. Studies show that regular Zoom users are more likely to pursue surgical and non-surgical procedures to improve their looks, all as a direct result of seeing themselves on a constant basis. Moreover, about one-third of all surveyed admitted to a "new appearance issue" which means they were distracted by something about their appearance that prior to the regular use of Zoom was not noticed or a bothersome issue.[6]

---

[6] Cristel, R., Demesh, D., & Dayan, S. (2020). Video conferencing impact on facial appearance: looking beyond the COVID-19 pandem-

Video platforms and parenting: The bad news regarding body image is that Zooming, FaceTime, Google Hangout, etc., is here to stay. In fact, we know that many employees have yet to return to their physical worksite at least full time and some may never do so. With schools, a couple outbreaks of a virus could shut things down and cause every aspect of learning to be online. This has (and will have) a direct impact on workers and students, and those who are young and vulnerable to body distortion have yet another barrier to hurdle.

For parents, the solution to Zooming is to encourage your child to turn off the image of themselves. I think it's that simple. When I emailed a student about an issue that would take about a minute, they responded with "Should we Zoom?" I snapped back with "Nope. Let's do that old fashion thing: A phone call." This little story demonstrates that these platforms are just the norm, and I get that. But your children's limiting the constant image of themselves is analogous to their limiting their use of social media: the less we engage in it and see ourselves, the less harm will be done.

ic. *Facial Plastic Surgery & Aesthetic Medicine, 22*(4), 238-239; Rice, S. M., Siegel, J. A., Libby, T., Graber, E., & Kourosh, A. (2021). Zooming into cosmetic procedures during the COVID-19 pandemic: the provider's perspective. *International Journal of Women's Dermatology, 7*(2), 213-216; Chandawarkar, A., Jenny, H., & Kim, R. (2021). Data-driven insights on the effects of COVID-19 on aesthetics: part I (passive analysis). *Aesthetic Surgery Journal, 41*(3), NP65-NP74.

Dolls and Action Figures

Despite the fact that it is years between the time that a child plays with dolls or action figures and the onset of a poor body image, some health professionals have theorized that figurines may be the single biggest factor in the battle for our children's minds. Taking a look at Barbie, Disney figurines, superheroes, and G.I. Joes from the perspective of this book can be an eye-opening experience. Think about it from this angle: many psychological problems that surface in adulthood can be attributed to our experience as children. With that in mind, how could we doubt the influence exerted on a child's developing brain by a distorted body like Barbie's? Holding, observing, dressing, and playing with these figurines, sometimes for years, must *somehow* play a role.

It's a cliché, but we're going to pick on Barbie as a contributing factor of body disorders in women. Did you know that in 1997 Mattel succumbed to public pressure by altering her measurements? They didn't change much because Barbie is still *far* from representing a normal woman's size. If Barbie were to be an adult, her size and dimensions would be as follows: Height - seven feet two inches, weight - 101 pounds, shoe size - five, and her breasts would fill an FF cup. And to add insult to injury, her waist would have the identical circumference of her head! It doesn't take an advanced degree in anatomy to know that Barbie suffers from a severe case of disproportionality. And, of course, Barbie's popularity has set the standard for many industry dolls.

Although it may be difficult for some to imagine, action figures have probably contributed to male body disorder in the same way that dolls have for girls. The authors of *The Adonis Complex* were the first to devote several pages to this phenomenon.[7] The modern-day versions of these toys (e.g., superheroes and even the *Star Wars* characters) are so muscular that the only difference between Superman and the world's largest steroid-bolstered bodybuilders is a cape, a mask, and colorful boots. In effect, these action figures reflect the growing pressures that young men deal with in magazines and the movies. The message they receive is loud and clear—the most desirable male body is one with bulging muscles, very little body fat, and virtually no body hair.

<u>Why dolls and action figures matter</u>: The detrimental effect that dolls and action figures have on the body issues of young men and women cannot be measured; it can only be theorized. But it is worth noting that it is nearly impossible for a girl or boy to avoid internalizing the drastic body shape and proportions of the toy they're playing with. Boys and girls play with figurines from the time they are young—sometimes before they can even talk. This may steer them toward a poor body image due to what is known as upward comparison (i.e., viewing something that is considered "ideal" like a male fitness model). Continually seeing and touching a doll that is beautiful, perfectly shaped, and forever young can only add to the milieu of body issues.

---

[7] Pope, H, Phillips, K., & Olivardia, R. (2000). The Adonis complex: the secret male crisis of male body obsession, The Free Press, New York.

Figurines and parenting: There are more choices than ever when it comes to purchasing toys for our kids, so understand that dolls and action figures are not the only option. It is important to note that all figurines should not be considered culpable, but we must be wise to the fact that many of them could be. Be smart about what you buy. Try to develop a healthy body image for your child while not compromising your morals or values. Many readers have told me that they have sent these plastic offenders off to other families via garage sales. But what's the message in that? Perhaps the positive spin is this: pass this information on to help guide or encourage a relative, friend, or toy-purchasing grandparent. Maybe we can do some little things to protect the fragile minds of the generations following our own.

Disney Princesses and Other Animated Heroes and Heroines

In my single days I couldn't name one female Disney character, let alone imagine the impact of these characters on an adolescent's body image. But marriage and having babies changed all of that. Recently on my daughter's fourth birthday, she was given a puzzle of Sophia, one of the many Disney princesses. For days straight, she asked me to help build this puzzle, and each time I was startled by two things: Sophia's huge eyes and tiny waist. I quickly estimated that her big, beautiful blue eyes were about seventy percent the size of her waist. Look for yourself; it's seventy percent. Even if her eyes were not as big as they were, it is impossible to ignore that her waist is a projected sixteen to eighteen inches. This is something you would only see on a pre-adolescent girl and rarely, if ever, on a woman.

I started to take a closer look at other Disney female lead characters found they were all the same: Cinderella, Jasmine (*Aladdin*), Belle (*Beauty and the Beast*), and even Snow White. Each one has more striking looks than the next and all have wildly out-of-proportion measurements. A Google search of these characters proved to be, excuse the pun, an eye-opening experience for sure. I also came across a set of images that placed Disney characters next to the real-life model they resembled. I immediately noticed how the real-life person looked so, um, normal. While these were clearly beautiful women that were being "compared" to the Disney characters, the differences in major facial and body characteristics were magnified as I shifted my gaze back and forth. And while each Disney character had a unique physical trait, they all shared qualities such as flowing hair, bright and full lips, a tiny waist, small feet, gorgeous (some might say seductive) eyes, and perfect youthful skin. So, in fairness to the real-life models, who *would* look and feel "normal" next to this?

And let's not forget the decades-long impact that animated characters may have had on boys also. For every female character, there's a male counterpart who is just as flawless as the female—big eyes, great hair, chiseled facial features, and muscular build. Just as male models and actors have increased in muscularity, so have animated male characters. Even Peter Pan has gently evolved in recent years from adolescence to a more physically appealing young man.

Why Disney and other animated characters matter: Just as we cannot precisely measure the "doll effect" on young men and women, the same is true for the effect of animated characters. But we can assume that an internalization of these images does occur on some level. You've seen how mesmerized your kids are when Disney's on the screen. The Disney folks are very good at what they do. Millions of children are exposed to these animated characters every day, often before they even learn to talk. So once again, it's probably safe to assume that such images play some role in developing their expectations of body image.

Animation and parenting: There are probably few dictums more controversial than telling parents to avoid all Disney movies, action figures, and related toys such as puzzles for four year-olds. I even have them in my own house. But just as with every other piece of information I offer, my goal is to raise a red flag. I want you to consider the impact that these things may be having on your child's well-being. Perhaps the answer to this potential problem is like so many discussed in this chapter—realize that while we may not completely escape from these factors, we can and should limit exposure to them.

Everyday Comments and Conversations

For unique reasons, one of the most difficult seasons of life is the teen years. During this time, comments about everything from your head to your toes seem to be fair game. Terms like "thigh gap," "thinspiration," and the ole standby of the disapproving "up and down" glance can leave an impression. I would venture to say that each person reading this probably has a vivid memory of how someone said or did something early in life that helped shape their body image, or at least had some degree of impact at the time. For a mature adult, most comments made by a middle or high school student would not even raise an eyebrow. But when you're young, the desire to be liked and accepted by peers is a priority, some would say a desperate need. It's been said that the pen is mightier than the sword and, in this case, we can include spoken words. Insults easily become injuries. Often injuries lead to action, sometimes an obsession. Other times, no action; just pain.

Why everyday conversations matter: In so many conversations among people, especially teenagers and children, there is very little thought about the hurt that words and comparisons may cause. One study showed that peer comparisons had greater impact on body dissatisfaction among female adolescents than social media and TV viewing.[8] And although there are a series of variables at work here, the result is almost universally the same. Picture one of your kids walking along the schoolyard fence, away from the confines of the classroom, and out of earshot of the principal. Maybe she doesn't have on the latest fashion (maybe you can't afford them) or perhaps her body is simply "normal." In an act of randomness as much as meanness, she becomes the target of thoughtless words. She's taunted, threatened, and ridiculed. What does she

---

[8] Ferguson, C., Munoz, M., Garza, A. & Galindo, M. (2014). Concurrent and Prospective Analyses of Peer, Television and Social Media Influences on Body Dissatisfaction, Eating Disorder Symptoms and Life Satisfaction in Adolescent Girls. *Journal of Youth & Adolescence, 43*, 1-14.

do? She can pretend not to care, but she will likely hold onto those comments for months or years to come. They can even become an internal compass of sorts, directing a constant inner-dialogue about her worth. Comparisons and insults put some people on the defensive and create angst in the heart that takes real grace to heal.

On the other hand, it is common for physical descriptors to reference physical beauty and weight. This is not problematic un-less it carries with it a critical or judgmental tone. We may not be able to stop adolescents and teens from gossiping, but as parents we can model something better. We can stop characterizing people based solely or primarily on their physical appearance. A parent who makes insulting comments about the looks and body weight of others is speaking volumes to their children. Two scenarios, both negative, are the result. First, such comments lead our chil-dren to believe that such language and tone is okay. Second, chil-dren will naturally begin to judge themselves by the standards you have created for others.

Everyday conversations and parenting: As parents, our role is to be positive examples of how to talk to and about those around us. We should strive to be sensitive to the good qualities of others when discussing things such as weight and beauty. We should nev-er emphasize or insinuate that beauty makes the individual more important or somehow assigns more dignity in God's eyes. It's good to be complimentary and acknowledge facial beauty and oth-er appealing physical characteristics as gifts from God. However, the more value we place on the outside, the less we focus on God's desire for each of us—a beautiful soul.

Cosmetic Surgery

William P. Adams, Jr., MD, and President of The Aesthetic Society said the following regarding the substantial increase in plastic surgery from 2020 to 2021: "Many factors have facilitated this growth including very high patient satisfaction, the pandemic and patients wanting to do something for themselves". Of course, it's for themselves. The notion that patients of plastic surgery were doing it for anyone but themselves seems was an 80s thing.

Each year, the Aesthetic Plastic Surgery Statistics (APSS) release pages of data that reflect trends within the industry and makes comparisons to previous years. The highlights of 2021 were:

- Americans spent over $14 billion on aesthetic procedures, the most ever;
- Overall procedures, surgical and non-surgical, were at an all-time high;
- Specialized face procedures (e.g. brow lift and facelift) increased 54% from 2020;
- Women accounted for 93% of the procedures;
- There are over 2,200 board certified plastic surgeons.[9]

Why cosmetic surgery matters: While most of the clients discussed here are women, it's obvious that men are feeling increasing pressure to improve themselves in ways that have long been more-

---

[9] The Aesthetic Society: The Statistics 2020-2021 (2022). Retrieved from https://cdn.theaestheticsociety.org/media/statistics/2021-TheAestheticSocietyStatistics.pdf

or-less exclusive to women. And considering that the numbers in-crease each year, the cosmetic surgery industry will not close its doors anytime soon. In fairness, a percentage of these procedures should not be viewed as major factors in our problem, nor should anyone feel bad about a procedure when the intent was corrective in nature. This may include replacement surgery (e.g., breast aug-mentation following mastectomy) or the removal of hair or age spots. But somewhere along this spectrum, the innocence of the action is no longer isolated to the person; it has an impact on those around us and the larger community as a whole.

Cosmetic procedures may contribute to body image problems for a couple of reasons. Making procedures appear to be more-or-less routine shifts the thinking about them. Once thought to be on-ly for those desperate to remain thin, appear young, etc., the pro-cedures are now increasingly thought to be helpful or necessary for anyone. Once desperation is no longer the motive, the extremes become normalized. It can artificially produce a feeling of "falling behind" if we don't do the same thing. When performing a facelift, the idea is to make the person look younger and more vibrant. If the surgery is successful, others may (and often do) feel some level of pressure to conform. While they may be the same age as the one who received the procedure, they no longer look as "youthful." In the end, an altered body is an extension of the Social Comparison Theory, which forces a comparison to something that is not natu-ral. The bottom line is this: God made us the way we are. Aging and everything that goes with it are part of his design.

Cosmetic surgery and parenting: It's probably best to point out early on that cosmetic surgery is a relatively common occurrence. It happens both in the world of actors and models, as well as for your neighbor and kid's teacher. I have heard from several different folks that these surgeries have become so common that they are often given out as gifts: a graduation gift to an eighteen-year-old daughter or a pick-me-up gift for a wife's fortieth birthday. This casual attitude towards such a serious medical procedure is extremely telling about how the cosmetic surgery industry has affected our culture.

A discussion with your age-appropriate child about cosmetic procedures would certainly raise awareness for them. It would also arm them with your opinions for when conversations with others arise. It all starts with you—the informed parent—realizing that magazines, social media, TV, movies, and just about everything else in this chapter propels the cosmetic surgery industry. Like many parents and teachers, I have found that one of the best conversation-starters is a newspaper article or TV news story that mentions cosmetic procedures. Follow up with a timely question, "What do you think about that?" Allow them to talk to you about their opinions and give them the benefit of yours, too.

Fitness Apparel and Athletes

On an annual basis, did you know that the only women's sport that receives more TV time than its male counterpart is beach volleyball? Anyone who has seen women's beach volleyball can quickly deduce why the men's game is not as popular. To put it bluntly,

it's because the women's attire— tiny bikinis worn by every player-
—provides more than one type of entertainment.

Not long ago, Sunday advertisement flyers for the local sports
store promoted sales for ordinary T-shirts and sneakers. Yet in the
last decade, a disproportionate amount of space has been dedicated
to tight-fitting, climate-negating sportswear. Each piece of clothing
seems to be designed so that low body fat and defined muscles are
prerequisites. Most of these products are true to their marketing
since they *can* improve performance. However, the average person
looking to participate in a sport or simply get some basic exercise is
not always looking for this apparel to yield gains in their performance. Not surprisingly then, this type of fitness apparel has become the norm, adding another avenue of pressure to look a certain way.

Competitive female athletes face additional challenges. It is well
documented that some coaches of particular sports (e.g., gymnas-
tics, ice skating, etc.) encourage their girls to become and remain
very lean to improve competitiveness. The standard attire has become so revealing that the female athlete has the added pressure to
look good and even appear sexy *while* competing. Therefore, it
should come as no shock that female athletes in aesthetic sports are
more prone to eating disorders than the general population or
among young women who participate in moderate exercise.[10]

---

[10] Krentz, E. M., & Warschburger, P. (2011). Sports-related correlates
of disordered eating in aesthetic sports. *Psychology of Sport & Exercise,*
12(4), 375-382.

Exercise physiologists have indeed determined a correlation between low body fat and improved performance for specific athletes such as gymnasts, figure skaters, volleyball players (beach or conventional), and those in track and field. While improved performance is a good thing, we must still take an honest look at the impact these clothes have. In all-too-many sports, the skimpy apparel has become the norm and even an expectation—not just at the level of the professional athlete but right down to the level of young children who engage in team and individual sports.

The fact is that we have the right to dress anyway we want. However, our rights need to be understood and implemented within a moral framework rooted in the dignity of the human person. Further, the church teaches that with every right there is responsibility.[11] It is important to understand that we are responsible for the way we dress, whether it is for informal situations, athletic competition, or employment. To overlook modesty is to contribute to the problem and directly ignore God's intention that the body be seen as an extension and reflection of him.[12]

Constant exposure to the issues addressed in this chapter can have a dual negative impact. They not only become a factor in how we judge ourselves, but also lead us to a life of being critical of others. It's harmful to lack appreciation of our own body, but the situation gets worse when we allow these factors to control how we see others, even our own family members.

---

[11] Catechism of the Catholic Church, No. 1914.
[12] 2/11/81 TB.

In the opening chapter, we talked about how we often forget or don't comprehend the body's purpose. Our increasingly secular culture is not prone to seeing the body as a good gift from God. When we fall in line, we tend to ignore the mind and soul that is attached to the body. And regardless of size and shape, each person has dignity and deserves respect as one created by God in his image. Christians with a vital relationship with God should aim to see every single person as one of his creations—beautifully and wonderfully made.

This chapter devoted some effort to identifying the triggers that lead to a poor body image, but such a discussion only addresses one small part of a bigger problem. The purpose of this book is to go beyond some of the causes to offer practical suggestions to help develop a healthy, realistic look at God's intentions for our bodies. Knowledge is power, and parents may have learned at least enough to create a long-term plan. With these tools, perhaps we can help our children leave a life of body obsession in the past.

And remember, don't let the media or anything else determine your worth. Let God do that.

Chapter 3

Did Mother Teresa Have Issues with Aging?
Girls, Women, and Body Image

To a great extent the level of any civilization is the level of
its womanhood. The higher her virtue, the more her character,
the more devoted she is to truth, justice, goodness,
the more a man has to aspire to be worthy of her.

— Archbishop Fulton J. Sheen

When I was a kid, I served as an altar boy in Detroit's second-oldest Catholic parish of Assumption Grotto. The church was beautifully appointed with dazzling stained-glass windows, ornate oak and teakwood ceiling beams, and neo-gothic chandeliers. As a boy, I was fascinated with every sight, sound, and smell that resonated within those consecrated walls. Between my brothers and me, we probably served over a thousand masses there, and I can still recall many of those moments in great detail. One memory has stuck with me over the years. It was during Communion. In those days, each parishioner received the Eucharist directly on his or her tongue at the altar rail, which meant that the altar boy was very up close and personal with everyone who accepted the host. And it always struck me as a bit odd when the older women approached and were dressed to the nines. We're talking heels and skirts, heavy rouge blush, make-up, lipstick, and *tons* of what we referred to as "old lady church perfume."

Most of these women were probably widows. They were well into their seventies and eighties—far beyond their dating and child-bearing years—yet they still wanted to look "presentable" to a discerning society. Perhaps a bit naively, I always wondered why.

Flash forward to just a few months ago and an interesting story a thirty-something woman told me about her middle school years. Every day, she rode the bus with the same students. One day, two of her male classmates simply blurted out, "Us [*sic*] guys agreed that you would be the prettiest girl in the class if you weren't fat." The unapologetic way those hurtful words were spoken shocked her, and she never forgot them. What was probably most surprising is that she wasn't fat or obese, just a few ticks to the wrong side of the scale. This woman was surely part of a growing number of nation-wide casualties of the "cheerleader effect" (the term I used in the previous chapter to refer to the problems that scantily clad women in the media cause as they pitch their cartoonish, pencil-thin bodies against those women of "normal" weight). It's a harsh comparison seeing that only a fraction of women have "modelesque" bodies. So, let's go back to our callous school bus guys. While many boys would have kept such thoughts to themselves, consider how many young girls—and all women for that matter—are silently judged in the same way each day they are seen in public.

Research clearly shows that a large percentage of females are dissatisfied with their bodies. Some studies indicate that as many as seventy percent suffer some degree of body distortion, with females in their teens and twenties regularly showing above fifty percent.[1] One study even revealed that while they decrease with age, body image concerns generally persist until old age[2]—just as they may have for those women who attended that wonderful old church back in Detroit. I choose to believe, however, that they were simply trying to please God rather than themselves or others.

What we do know is that for many, maintaining a healthy body image is an ongoing and frustrating fight. And it's not just an American phenomenon. Women in other advanced societies such as Korea, Australia, and Great Britain have higher rates of poor body image than their counterparts in poorer countries.[3] In most

---

[1] Cash, T., Morrow, J., Hrabosky, J., & Perry, A. (2004). How has body image changed? a cross sectional investigation of college women and men from 1983 to 2001. *Journal of Consulting and Clinical Psychology, 72,* 1081-1090; Vartanian, L., Giant, C., & Passino, R. (2001). Ally McBeal vs. Arnold Schwarzenegger: Comparing mass media, interpersonal feedback and gender as predictors of satisfaction with body thinness and muscularity. *Social Behavior and Personality, 29,* 711–724.

[2] Quittkat, H. L., Hartmann, A. S., Düsing, R., Buhlmann, U., & Vocks, S. (2019). Body dissatisfaction, importance of appearance, and body appreciation in men and women over the lifespan. *Frontiers in Psychiatry, 10,* 864.

[3] Jung, J. & Forbes, G. (2007). Body dissatisfaction and disordered eating among college women in China, South Korea, and the United States: contrasting predictions from sociocultural and feminist theories, *Psychology of Women Quarterly, 31*(4), 381-393; Sheffield, J., Tse, K. & Sofronoff, K. (2005). A comparison of body-image dissatisfaction and eating disturbance among Australian and Hong Kong women, *European Eating Disorders Review, 13* (2)112-124; Grogan, S. (2021). Body image:

underdeveloped countries, of course, the focus is on meeting some pretty basic needs—clean water, eating something other than fish head stew with rotted rice, and fundamental health care. These aren't the types of folks who are going to give a hoot about weight gain or attaining a certain "look." In the United States, for example, being tanned and thin suggests being in control and affluent. The irony is that, in present times, plumpness in many of regions of the world signals wealth, health, and prosperity.[4] Consider the women in these poor regions—what do you suppose they would think to hear of the developed world's eating disorders and the obsession with being thin? They probably feel those stories are exaggerated or even untrue. And what would they think of the prevalence of gastric bypass surgery?

Our country has developed a certain degree of madness in this area. The average citizen in America has so much in comparison to people in other nations that it has caused us to desire the unattainable. Teens want a BMW for their first car, women and men want to look like Barbie and Ken, and we're obsessed with youth. I understand that it is good for societies, and individuals for that matter, to strive to be better. But we have lost our way when we have convinced ourselves that *having and being more* is better than *being better.* And we have really lost our way when people react more strongly against someone who aspires to stay true to personal reli-

---

understanding body dissatisfaction in men, women and children, London/New York, Routledge.

   [4] Rothblum, E. (1990). "Women and weight: fad or fiction, *The Journal of Psychology*, 124, 5-24.

gious beliefs than against someone who has dozens of surgeries because she aspires to become a "real life Barbie."

But, I digress. Let's take a closer look at a timeline on body types.

Desiring thinness and muscularity in western culture is a relatively new phenomenon. For much of our country's history, middle and upper class men would shun tanned and thin women. They thought of them as the working class or outdoor type, even peasants, and thus not desirable. The same was certainly true in other affluent regions. However, in the early 1900s, the United States moved from a rural farming culture to an industrialized nation, and a different mentality began to emerge. As a direct result, physicians in the 1920s advocated that women become more conscious of weight gain since higher body fat on women was thought to be "energy depleting." They suggested that being overweight was less than desirable for a growing, more sophisticated society.[5]

Those gentle comments from doctors on obesity (a comparatively small matter at the time) and the growing distribution of fashion magazines can be linked to the frenzy we see today. In fact, it was during this period that women's magazines went from using pencil drawings to depict the latest clothing trends to color photographs. And like the slick images of today, such publications began to have a strong effect on the female reader's own body image.[6]

---

[5] Gordon, R. (1990). Anorexia and bulimia: anatomy of a social epidemic, Oxford, Blackwell.

[6] Orbach, S. (1993). Hunger strike: the anorexic's struggle as a metaphor for our age, London, Penguin.

Then came that newfangled entity known as the talking motion picture. Movies had an influence that can hardly be overstated. The movie viewer of the 1930s and 1940s could not help but notice a change from the slender actress of the silent movie era to the more curvaceous look of screen performers such as Mae West and Lana Turner. Because these advances in motion pictures were all new and powerful in their own way, they had quite an impact. Seeing the shapely film stars in volumes of color photographs probably swayed that generation in ways similar to how media sways young women today.

In the late 1950s, the "sweater" models such as Marilyn Monroe, Jane Russell, and Jayne Mansfield became popular, and never did the country see such a stir over a specific body type. It was impossible for it to go unnoticed! They all were pretty with large breasts and relatively small waists. In essence, this was the birth of today's desire for the Barbie-doll look.

And something else happened earlier in that same decade. In 1953, a then-unknown Marilyn Monroe posed for the first issue of *Playboy* magazine. The editor of *Playboy* purposely omitted the date on the cover of that first issue since he was unsure whether there would be a second one. Little did he know. Even though the world had seen nudes in pictorials and paintings for centuries, it could be argued that this magazine single-handedly altered public opinion about naked women. Nudity was no longer isolated to art or underground dirty magazines—it went mainstream.

Playboy led the charge for its readers to admire a woman's body for pleasure alone and purportedly did so in a "classy" and somehow acceptable way. Many still argue that the magazine never has been classy or acceptable. Other male magazines such as to-day's *Maxim* and *Men's Health* have not so slowly nudged *Playboy* aside. In a way, they provide the same service to their mostly male readership by sandwiching the provocative photos of women be-tween legitimate articles about investing and workout tips.

Very clever, but they're not reinventing the wheel.

The effect that *Playboy*, *Maxim's* "Girl of the Week" or *Men's Health's* "Top 10 Hottest Actresses" have on male readers has con-tributed to the same problem. Subconsciously or not, men make known their expectations and desires for all women to be sexy, well-built, and attractive. As a result, negative body issues develop-ing in girls shift into hyper-speed and rarely slow down. Simply put, women *know* that men desire those "photoshopped" beauties and, out of their natural need to be wanted, they will strive for that same perfection. Suddenly, parents see a change in their sweet and caring adolescent girl who once played dress-up and danced in adorable recitals. She becomes a frustrated teenager who is ob-sessed with every detail of her life that doesn't fit a certain mold—especially with perceived imperfections of her body.

One of the few upsides to the current state is that men don't wish for or expect women to be nearly as perfect as women *think* they should be.[7] The downside is that the standards for beauty and

---

[7] Huon, G. Sue E. Morris, S. & Brown, L. (1990). Differences between male and female preferences for female body size, *Australian Psycholo-gist, 25*, (3) 314 – 317; Bergstrom, R., Neighbors, C. & Lewis, M. (2004). Do men find "bony" women attractive?: Consequences of misperceiving

perfection are still high, and they are having an obvious and damaging impact on girls and women of all ages and ethnicities. A simple reflection back to the barely-overweight girl who was unfairly called fat demonstrates the pressure that women feel from others. And they pressure themselves as well. Either way, the anxiety is very real, and it's as much a part of a girl's everyday life as choosing outfits or changing hairstyles.

Even though the men in a woman's social circle may be culpable to a degree, a young, confused woman may be her own worst enemy. She probably has trouble avoiding the triggers that create such perfectionistic standards. As parents, we cannot imagine our blossoming daughters saying to themselves, "Hey, these fashion magazines and risqué TV-shows are harming me." But the truth is, they *are* causing damage. They heighten women's frustration and anxiety about their own bodies even as they fuel their competitive side. For some, the need to compete is so fierce that they evaluate themselves based not just on how many men they attract, but on how many or how well they attract men *away* from other women. While the solution may not be fully realized by turning off the TV or putting down a magazine, it wouldn't be a bad place to start.

So, why has obtaining a positive body image become such a difficult and complex issue for women? It appears that the need to have a flawless body stems from a distinctive combination of social, health, and economic factors (many of which were discussed in the previous chapter). But professionals point to another major culprit:

---

opposite sex perceptions of attractive body image, *Body Image, 1*, 183-191.

women cling to the illusion that they can (or must) have it all. They have become convinced that they should be able to work, be socially active, raise children, be a great spouse, *and* be perfectly attractive all at the same time. Just the thought of it is exhausting . . . and impossible. Yet as most of us know when we try to gain it all, it is inevitable that something (or everything) will be lost in the process. Just remember what our wise old mothers once told us: when you try to please everyone, you end up pleasing no one.

Least of all, ourselves. Or God.

Often, trying to have it all and be it all leads to a feeling of being out of control. And when all these pressures converge on women, some respond with a need to master one of the few things that *can* be controlled: you guessed it, the body.[8]

Therefore, the woman's feeling of helplessness can be remedied if this feeling of being "in-control" can be regained. This is where the intense desire to be (or stay) thin and attractive fully kicks in. Moreover, women learn from an early age that unattractiveness and an unhealthy body weight is associated with unhappiness, laziness, lack of discipline, and lower self-confidence. And all of these are perceived as harmful when trying to land a good job, find a good mate, or establish friendships with influential people.

Nevertheless, women's values have been so distorted that many consider thinness to be the highlight of all accomplishments. At best, adolescent and teenage girls are just a few steps behind. This

---

[8] Grogan, (2021); Bordo, S. (1993). Unbearable weight: feminism, Western Culture, and the body, University of California Press, Berkeley, California.

certainly seemed to be the case of the college woman in this chapter's opening paragraphs. Everything she said indicated that her overall contentment in life was controlled by the amount of fat on her body.

How many times have we heard a woman say (aloud or by their facial expression) that she "hates" a pretty, slender woman who walks by? She doesn't *really* hate her—she's just envious. She sees the thin woman as in-control, happy, and worry-free. She probably even wonders how the woman remains so impossibly tiny despite the ever-availability of appetizing foods. Further, a woman's obsession with her body does not stop and start with being slender. Worrying about her hip measurement, breast size, hair (color, style, and length), height, leg and derrière-shape, posture, feet attractiveness, eye color, makeup schemes, skin tone (take a deep breath, this could take a while), teeth alignment, waistline measurement, glasses style, facial and underarm hair, neckline length and firmness, muscle firmness (but not masculinity), eyebrows size and shape, jewelry choices, fashion sense that includes trendy accessories, poutiness of lips, and gracefulness of hands all add to the craziness.

With all of this considered, it is vital that we take a stab at healing this monumental issue. So, let's go back to the beginning—the real beginning in the Garden of Eden. Let's continue discussing, as we did in the first chapter, what all this has to do with a headlong divorce from the Truth. Saint John Paul II tells us that we became detached from the true meaning of the body because of the fall. In the beginning, Adam and Eve were naked without shame. They both understood the meaning of the body and recognized it as a gift. And since there was no sin or shame, Adam and Eve saw the body as God intended it, as pure and good.[9] Eve did not see herself as imperfect, nor did any conflict arise about the shape, size, and uniqueness of her body.

But the Garden of Eden, where humanity began, is also where body distortion began. Although God's plan for man, as represented by the body, is to unite us to himself and to each other, it is obvious that Satan had his own plan. His plan was and remains to be a divider—between people, and between God and us.[10] When Satan's plan is successful, we are critical of those around us and of ourselves, regardless of how we *really* look. Since God created women to be naturally attracted to men (and vice versa), there's a crisis when the woman does not see herself as attractive or neglects in some way to see her body as inherently good.

Genesis 3:16 reads, "Your urge shall be for your husband, and he shall be your master." Perhaps this explains why a woman can see herself as unworthy. It has been suggested that this verse describes a woman's fear of being alone and unwanted, as well as her need to be physically appealing to men. By itself, the woman's craving to be desired is understandable. We all need human contact, and all want to be loved. But these natural needs become problematic when they are combined with a woman's poor body image and lead to (sometimes extreme) efforts to ensure that she captures the attention of the man across the room. Consider the women who have numerous sex partners or dress provocatively to validate

---

[9] 1/7/80 TB.
[10] Catechism of the Catholic Church, No. 394.

themselves as worthy. And as we will continue to discuss, such preoccupation leads to a host of unhealthy behaviors that keep us from building a stronger relationship with God.

The Great Deceiver is aware of our need to grow closer to God. He is well pleased when we sabotage ourselves by turning something as innocent and good as being healthy and fit into an obsession. Fitness magazines and health club ads have done their own part to cloud the difference between "be healthy" and "be perfect." When the line between these two is blurred, confusion sets in.

Some advertisers pride themselves on trying to promote health and fitness, but bombard the consumer with comments about obtaining the perfect body. Most of us realize that perfection is not possible, nor does it correlate to our physical health. We can be very healthy and fit and not meet any of today's criteria for perfection. Let's go back to the crowded grocery store with the magazine covers that mention the word "health" or "fitness" directly next to the phrase "Build the Dream Body" or "Get Picture Perfect Abs." Stand in line long enough, and it's easy to see how someone would start to believe that this is truth—*and* the way to proverbial happiness. Many young women who through a habitual exercise routine, disciplined dieting, or just good genetics, already have a trim physique seem to worry as much about maintaining their figure as others do in trying to achieve one. This confusion may help explain the millions of women who suffer from eating disorders. When we fail to see the difference between being healthy and being perfect, we fail to see God's intention for us.

Our faith, and particularly our former pope, has been so helpful in this regard. Saint John Paul II directly addressed the need to fully embrace God's plan for the body when he said, "Man cannot live without love. He remains a being that is incomprehensible for himself, his life is senseless, if love is not revealed to him, if he does not encounter love, if he does not experience it and make it his own, if he does not participate intimately in it."[11] The pope stresses this because striving for the "dream body" has become a preoccupation for too many young women. Many parents have stood by feeling helpless as they witnessed this preoccupation taking their daughters further and further away from our real purpose of loving.

Regardless of how God is calling us to serve him, it requires the physical body. Saint Paul tells us that offering our body for service to others is a spiritual act of worship: "I urge you therefore, brothers, by the mercies of God, to offer your bodies as a living sacrifice, holy and pleasing to God" (Rom 12:1). When we become willing to die to this perfection affliction, as Christ died for us, we begin to fulfill the real purpose for our existence. The young woman mentioned earlier in this chapter is like many others: she feels the meaning of her existence is closely tied to how well she meets the standards of the physically perfect woman. Unless we shift our desire from achieving perfection in the eyes of others, to a desire to be seen perfect in God's loving eyes, the pursuit of bodily perfection will remain an affliction.

Sometimes, I think back to Detroit's East Side, and those tired old souls who attended Assumption Grotto Church when I was just a kid. If I had been older, more insightful, and less shy, I might have wanted to approach them. I wish I had the wisdom then to tell

---

[11] Saint John Paul II, Encyclical Letter, 4/10/79.

them that God has a wonderful plan, and it's the reason for his incarnation, passion, and resurrection. But, you know, they probably already knew that. I further wish I could have thanked them for presenting themselves so nicely to our Lord.

Consider this by Saint Jerome: "Either we must speak as we dress, or dress as we speak. Why do we profess one thing and display another? The tongue talks of chastity, but the whole body reveals impurity."

Many women and young girls today may come to Mass with the intention of being prayerful, but they fail in some way since the norms and expectations of society have shifted, even for Mass. It seems that for some, Sunday at church is a contest for "Who's the most sexy?" or worse, "Who can come to Mass and *not* get kicked out due to inappropriate attire?" We've all seen such inappropriate and immodest dress. It's one of the sure ways to offend God who is the only appropriate focus of attention at Mass. If a young woman fails to see this, it's the duty of mom and dad to have a good, old-fashioned sit-down with her. Society is already inundated with too much skin and the oversexualization of women in general. For heaven's sake, let's do our best to keep it out of Mass.

Further, don't forget what a young woman's attire can do to the men and boys who are trying desperately to have a wholesome and holy hour with God. The distraction of immodest dress, especially during holy Mass, works to shift our focus from Christ. And he is the very one who promises that we can be restored to our original glory, be without shame, and live in peace with our bodies, others, and God.[12]

And remember; don't let the media or anything else determine your worth. Let God do that.

---

[12] 1/9/80 TB.

Chapter 4

Did Saint John Paul II Consider Testosterone Injections?

Men, Boys, and Body Image

We should love the body insofar as
it is obedient and helpful to the soul,
since the soul, with the body's help and service,
is better disposed for the service and
praise of our Creator and Lord.

—Saint Ignatius

In 1995, New York Yankee pitcher Jim Abbott threw a brilliant no-hitter. This is no small accomplishment—less than 300 pitchers in history have done it. And we're talking as far back as 1876. But Abbott's feat was an even bigger accomplishment because he was born without a fully developed right arm and hand.

That bears repeating . . . the man was a major league pitcher and has only *one hand.*

Jim's a lefty, so here's how he would do it: After catching the ball with the mitt on his left hand, he would cradle the glove under his right arm and grab the baseball with his left. Then he would deliver the next pitch and, as part of his follow-through, would slip his left hand into the glove in preparation for the return ball— either a batted ball or one returned from the catcher. The entire sequence was fascinating to watch. But he did it seamlessly, thousands of times in his eight-year major league career and in the countless games prior to the big leagues. In fact, if you catch yourself with a few extra moments, go to YouTube and check it out. You'll be humbled at the engineering marvel that is the human body and spirit.

Quite an athlete, Jim was not only a dominating pitcher in high school, but he was the winning pitcher in the 1988 gold medal game in the Olympics in Seoul. He also played quarterback at a major high school that made it to the state playoffs and was known to be a respectable basketball player. He wanted nothing more than to be recognized for his athletic ability but could never forget his handicap since he was so often reminded that he was born without a right hand.

Following Abbott's baseball career, his five-year old daughter asked him to come to her school to be a part of "Daddy Career Day." He delayed saying yes; probably thinking that since he was no longer a major league pitcher, he had no career to talk about. But he wanted to please his daughter, figured it was another opportunity to educate and inspire others regarding his disability, and so he went. He answered a couple of random questions like, "Do you have a dog?" and, "Is your house big?" But then he fielded one from a little girl seated in the first row and beaming. She asked him if he loved his little hand. Abbott hesitated but answered that he did. That question came from his daughter.

Now Abbott has been through a lot due to his missing hand. You probably know from your own kids that elementary school hasn't changed much over the decades. You can bet that when Abbott was young, he certainly took relentless teasing from his classmates. And the whispers and stares continued into adulthood. Although he experienced immense success at literally every level of baseball, he was rarely spared the scrutiny and undesired attention that disabled persons regularly confront. But he's always said, "I still love my 'little hand.'" Oh, how this must please God.

One of the reasons that Abbott embraced being a major leaguer is that it created opportunities for him to meet and talk to disabled children while they were seeking his autograph. Getting an autograph was often the last thing the kids wanted. Most of them just wanted to see their hero up close and talk to a person who succeeded at what so many little boys dream of—being a star at the highest level of sport. Despite uneasiness about his hand, Abbott made sure that he passed on what his parents instilled in him, which was to persevere and focus on the gift that God had granted him. Many would logically assume that his gift was his major league talent. But his real gift was that he loved himself—bad hand and all—and knew that he had been given the greatest gift of all: life.

It must be quite a challenge for a parent to teach a child who is disabled or diseased to appreciate and even love his or her body. This takes a lot of encouragement, compassion, and faith-filled investment from people that care about them, especially during the early years. Other parents have children who are not actually disabled but are not healthy and fit. Their task is challenging, too. In fact, it might be safe to say that parents (faithful or not) with physically challenged children have developed effective language to help their children appreciate what their bodies *can* do rather than what they *can't*. In his book, *Imperfect: An Improbable Life*, Abbott doesn't provide many specifics on how his parents helped him overcome his disability other than providing regular encouragement and motivation to stay determined. In reading his book, however, I sense that Abbott is a lot like most of us: confident in some situations and vulnerable in others. The irony of being born with no abnormalities is that it might subtly increase the inclination to work toward bodily perfection, simply because it seems attainable.

Clothing companies, the cosmetics industry, videos, television programs, and others have long targeted girls, making them insecure about themselves. Now boys have giant bulls-eyes drawn on *their* backs, too. We can almost see company executives maniacally wringing their hands, saying: "Ya know, we can get our pound of flesh from them, too!" Even if we're aware of the barrage of ads geared toward our tweens, we tend to shrug off the men's body spray, shaving gels, and hair care commercials with more than a glance. Yet they are saying the same things to our sons that have long been designated for our daughters: they need better teeth and hair, and their bodies are not perfect! This warrants our concern and concerted attention. Boys are vulnerable, too. They account for half the teen marketplace—a fact that did not slip by advertising executives unnoticed. In case parents out there have missed this, boys now have become twice as particular about the way they dress, how they style their hair, and even shave their bodies than did their counterparts in, say, the WWII generation. And it's all based on the same motivating fears that teenage girls have: be well groomed and have the perfect body or be shunned by your peers as if you have a disease. Many parents wait too late to address the issues of excessive grooming product purchases, sports supplements, and workouts. Don't wait. It's always good to have discussions regarding any aspect of health. By the late teens, habits may be ingrained and it may be difficult to make an impact. Sadly, as with so many conversations with our children, those meant to counteract the effects of the advertising industry on our sons should take place a year or two before we think they should.

And, as many know, there has been suspected steroid use by athletes in a variety of sports—track and field, cyclists, and tennis, not to mention the standards of football and baseball. Well, actually, it's been more than suspected use. Many athletes (some of them heroes to our youth) have actually been convicted of using anabolic steroids. But steroid use is not limited to athletes or serious bodybuilders. The shocker is that many students have admitted that they do this *not* for performance enhancement, but simply to look better.[1] Surprising, huh? But it does indicate that extreme measures are taken to look like a magazine model or ripped actor.

And consider this: how many high schoolers *wish* to take steroids but can't afford them, or simply don't know how to obtain them? Muscle-building products, in addition to anabolic steroids and human growth hormones, continue to grow in sales. And we

---

[1] Kanayama, G., & Pope Jr, H. G. (2018). History and epidemiology of anabolic androgens in athletes and non-athletes. *Molecular and cellular endocrinology, 464*, 4-13; Sandvik, M. R., Bakken, A., & Loland, S. (2018). Anabolic–androgenic steroid use and correlates in Norwegian adolescents. *European Journal of Sport Science, 18*(6), 903-910.

haven't even broached protein supplements, amino acids, and nitric oxide, which are readily available almost everywhere, affordable, and legal. The manufacturers of all these products have widened their audience to include teens. And we know what that means. If teens are attracted to it, adolescents will take note, and so on.

Until recently, parental concerns for their children's body image were dominated by concern for their daughters. Their sons, on the other hand, were taught from a young age to stay focused on a couple of basic sociological principles: to provide a financially and physically stable environment for those around them. In other words, "Be a man." But pressures from outside sources that have plagued women for years are now at work to redefine what a man is. Today's advertising culture is telling us that a man is defined by his overall physical attractiveness, sexuality, and stamina. And, oh yeah, he should also do the things that make him a good family guy.

Not too long ago, boys would daydream about being comic book heroes and sports stars. And as adults, it was common for men to adopt role models that more realistically defined manhood. In our parents' and grandparents' time, actors such as Cary Grant, Jimmy Stewart, and John Wayne were conventional male icons. They had a no-nonsense attitude and always seemed to do the right thing. Today, the defining characteristics of a man are not as clear. It's quite possible that the question, especially given the current confusion on sex and gender, "What is manhood?" would be answered in as many different ways as the number of people asked.

Because media figures and actors with bulging muscles have become far more common in the last decade or so, the playing field has changed. The qualifications of manhood have broadened, and the standard has gotten a lot tougher to meet. That is, men may or may not have to be emotionally strong and financially secure, but the unspoken requirement of meeting a certain physical standard seems always to be lurking. While slender, muscular bodies have been idealized since the Roman Empire, those standards haven't had much of an impact on today's man for many years. It's a different game now. For the first time in history, men have become extremely conscious of their looks—and they are repeatedly being told that they should be.

Until recently men have not experienced serious pressure to look a certain way from any real outside source. This notable shift may have started with popular movies in the 1980s when actors such as Sylvester Stallone and Arnold Schwarzenegger stumbled into nearly every scene with bigger-than-average muscles, extremely low body fat, and no body hair. While Schwarzenegger and Stallone graced the big screen shirtless many times, their characters were not so threatening to the youth of their day. They were more like buffoonish action-figures coming to life. Not many took them as serious sex symbols that appealed to either gender on a mass level.

However, Brad Pitt in the 1991 movie *Thelma and Louise* may have single-handedly changed things. He appears to be the first male actor in motion picture history whose brief role will be remembered more for his looks (and body) than for his acting. In the bedroom scene, Pitt's toned body was so much the focus that it stunned some viewers. Many movie critics agreed that this was something never really experienced by movie audiences until that point. At least not with a man as the focus. The fact that Pitt's character was portrayed as a sexual object was offensive to some but made others drool. The women who found this characterization, uh, appealing, could hardly help but make flattering comments about his body. Such comments overheard by (or said directly to) men, would surely add to a man's anxiety over not being in better shape.

Also in the 1990s, mainstream magazines began to slowly undress their male models, featuring them in nude or semi-nude pictorials. Women's fashion magazine readers had seen this for years, but it soon became the norm for male readers to see another male as more than a "pretty face." Their shirts came off (literally) and male readers became increasingly self-conscious about their own bodies. In addition, *Playgirl* magazine, as the authors of the book *The Adonis Complex* assert, had its own influence on men's body issues. By applying a specific formula to the male models from mid-1970s to the late 1990s, the authors have determined that they became progressively more muscular *and* displayed a lower percentage of body fat. On those same models, since the 1970s there's also been a difference in body hair (less of it) and age (they are younger).[2]

---

[2] Pope, H, Phillips, K., Olivardia, R. (2000). The Adonis complex: the secret male crisis of male body obsession, The Free Press, New York.

These days, boys and young men are exposed to so many images of ripped models and actors and even professional bodybuilders that it's hard to keep track. Consider alone the countless number of movies about superheroes, in which the bodies of the characters may have been perfected by computers. At the least, the actors tell tales of intense workouts and strict dieting months prior to filming. Reality or not, kids fall for the look. Further, chiseled bodies have become so much a part of our daily intake that no one blinked an eye when a female reality show star said steroids "make guys bigger, and better looking." Talk about upping the ante. Her statement about steroids parallels a now-famous comment by Sylvester Stallone: "I like my girlfriends to be anorexic-ly thin." I remember a female writer saying that Stallone's remark was so powerful that it will take decades to calm women's general fears about their bodies. Why the press didn't pull a similar alarm on the comments about guys and steroids is unknown. But you can bet that these comments and others like them are here to stay.

What does this mean for a boy today? Everything.

Men and boys are experiencing the strain to reach a certain level of attractiveness of both face *and* body, a clear change from the standard desire to be handsome, rugged, or suave. Now the standard includes sexy. The over-sexualization of boys has gained a lot of traction in recent years. I've never seen the numbers, but my guess is that posing sexually in a selfie is nearly as common for guys as it is for girls. I remember seeing sporting goods store mannequin dressed in the now-requisite tight fitting dry-fit shirt. The mannequin's chest and arms looked like those of Hercules. Given today's atmosphere, *that* didn't surprise me. What did surprise me was the mannequin didn't look a day over sixteen years old.

Boys' minds become clouded with everything from teenage vampires and werewolves with great pecs, to ads for T-shirts so tight that they would seem snug on an adolescent. And it doesn't help when young girls flaunt their shapely bodies via selfies and reality shows, either. Naturally, the boys will think that the only way to get a beautiful girl's attention is to be the male equivalent. All of this has led to a rising number of men who are unhappy with their bodies. Yeah, like thirty-three percent of us. Although this is still a much lower number than the fifty to seventy percent (depending on the study being quoted) for women, it's drastically higher than the ten percent noted in the 1970s.[3]

It is also evident that the media has made the same impact on men as it has on women—it just took them a little longer. As with the models in *Playgirl*, males in other magazines and on TV have become younger, more muscular, and have decreased in body fat. It has given rise to a reversal (of sorts) of anorexia, known as "bigorexia" or muscle dysmorphia. Just as a woman may never see herself as thin, many young men feel that, despite being in really good shape, they still don't look good enough. An example, albeit an extreme one, may best be seen in champion bodybuilders, who are not just muscularly built, but are downright enormous.

This all reverts back to an issue already touched upon: fear. More than ever before, men (and now boys) are growing in fear

---

[3] Grogan, S. (2021). Body image: understanding body dissatisfaction in men, women and children, London/New York, Routledge.

that they cannot be successful, handsome, or even a "regular guy" unless they look a certain way or achieve a particular body type. And who's easier to scare into thinking they're not up to par than a young person?

A frightening example of how fear seems to reign in many situations can be gleaned from the increased interest in steroids. Despite all the information on the dangers of using steroids, our young men still use (or want to use) them. The great harbinger's voice out there has fallen on deaf ears. It seems the need for some men to meet a certain muscular standard outweighs the inherent risks of taking steroids. If this sounds like a public service announcement, it is.

The Bible states, "Do not conform any longer to the pattern of this world but be transformed by the renewing of the mind" (Rom 12:2). Hmmm, it's almost like God saw the future. Steroid users are willing to take their chances, or worse yet, may not even care about the negative outcomes. I remember one conversation in which a student confided to me that he wanted to take steroids. He was an ordinary guy, not an athlete or an avid bodybuilder. I reminded him of the countless side-effects *and* that they are illegal, but all he wanted to know about was their effectiveness. We were like two ships passing in the night.

Though more subtle than steroid use, the use of men's cosmetic products has risen substantially, especially in the past decade. The next time you're watching a televised sporting event, take note of what's playing during commercial time. It's loud and clear. While there is nothing wrong or immoral with appropriate grooming or hygiene (or sound nutrition and fitness plans, for that matter), the voices are all working to point men in the same direction. Men and boys are becoming increasingly more preoccupied with their looks to the point that it may be bordering on an obsession.

Again, this preoccupation is not new. It began in the Garden of Eden. Prior to the serpent making his presence known, there was peace and harmony there. It was a place where Adam and Eve saw everything that God made, including their bodies, and agreed that all of it was good. Adam would even likely agree that physical activity is also good for the body. Engaging in an exercise regimen can reflect that we care for the body God has given us and realize we can benefit from rewards that it brings. We can experience and enjoy an increase in energy, a strong heart, and better sleep patterns—all noble goals.

This is good, right?

Yes, it is, but we cannot expect perfection. Our aim should be to associate exercise with developing a healthy, even attractive body in compliance with the Lord's desire for us to be happy. A healthy contentment should lead to awareness that a pursuit for perfection is nothing more than a thinly disguised form of gluttony. Rather, we should look to employment, physical activity, sports, recreation, and hobbies as ways to live a fuller life and to glorify God (1 Cor 6:20). Yes, we please God when we score a touchdown, get a base hit, or reach a new maximum bench press— as long as we accomplish the goal in an ethical manner *and* acknowledge God as the creator of this fine machine called the body. Actually, many athletes get this. Recall the number of occasions that you've heard an athlete thank God immediately after they have contributed to a big win.

Also, recognizing the body as being willed into existence by God is one of the ways that we can acknowledge God's love. It is virtuous to be thankful for the opportunities he gives us. Failing to see that the body is God's instrument for the message of salvation is failing to see the very reason we were given life.[4]

Adam would agree with Saint Paul who said that taking care of the body is wise since it houses the Holy Spirit (1 Cor 6:19). If body obsession had been an issue in the Garden, it would have firmly corrected the wrong thinking. Before the fall, Adam would have taken care of his body for all the right reasons. He would not have abused it or become absorbed with it in any way (including taking steroids!). Further, any man untainted by original sin would have realized that too much time spent on perfecting the body would be futile. Let's leave perfection to God and, instead, spend more time investigating our real purpose of life, which is to constantly ask, "How can I serve the Lord today?"

Once Adam sinned, however, his purpose and mentality changed. God told him that "by the sweat of your face, shall you get bread to eat" (Gen 3:19), indicating that Adam must now labor for his food and fight for his very existence. From that moment forward, man became a hunter and gatherer. In addition to being responsible for providing for his family, he would now have to function as their protector.

---

[4] 2/20/80 TB.

In fact, despite the technological and social advances that the world has experienced, the man is still considered by many as the traditional head of the household. Caring for his wife and children entails many responsibilities—feeding, defending, providing spiritual guidance, and many other duties that demand strength and stamina. So, for a variety of reasons, the man *should* be strong. But nowhere is it written that the man needs a flawless body to farm effectively or that he must have a full head of hair to tend to his family. It's not necessary, that is, to be physically perfect to earn a good wage, to be an adoring husband, or to be a loving father. Thankfully, God created us to be inclined to do what is good, and if certain distractions are limited, our souls can remain wholesome. Our role is to nurture the inclination toward the good by seeking out his will.

And remember, don't let the media or anything else determine your worth. Let God do that.

Chapter 5

What if We Only Got Today
What We Prayed for Yesterday

I will go peaceably and firmly to the Catholic Church: for if Faith is so important to our salvation, I will seek it where true Faith first began, seek it among those who received it from God Himself.

—Saint Elizabeth Ann Seton

One night as my wife Alecia was putting our then four-year-old daughter Clare to bed, Alecia started talking about the Holy Trinity. She told Clare, "There's God the Father, God the Son – Jesus, and God the Holy Spirit." Referring to the final comment, Clare said, "God's a bird?" One comment like that puts teaching a kid about God into perspective. Many aspects of religion and faith can be challenging for adults and difficult for children—especially Catholic teaching which is rich in theology and philosophy. But as many of us have come to learn, most of the burden of teaching the Faith is placed on us, the parents. We have to weave as many stories, parables, and examples of how to build a relationship with God as we can. And, at some point, usually when our babies go off to college, we have to rely on what we've taught them and implore the Holy Spirit to offer constant guidance.

One of the most difficult concepts to pass on to kids is that God often appears to us in ways that seem non-eventful, even mundane.

But he *is* there, always reaching his hand to us while our responsibility is to reach back. Sometimes, Catholicism gets a bad rap, and some of those critics are ones who call themselves faithful to its teachings. But how many of those who are negative toward the Catholic faith have never really put it to practice? In fact, the late Archbishop Fulton Sheen said, "There are not one hundred people in the United States who hate The Catholic Church, but there are millions who hate what they wrongly perceive the Catholic Church to be."

The Catholic Church is known for its teaching, also known as the Catechism. The teaching is rich, well-explained, well-reasoned, and offered to us daily to provide significance to our life. But still, it is up to us parents to engage it, embrace it, and pass it on to our kids so that we provide a fighting chance for them to lead a faith-filled life.

One of the common, painful experiences of many parents is witnessing the failure of a child to meet his or her potential in any aspect of life. But when we have children who fail to see or accept God's grace—which many of us see it as the core to a fulfilled life—it can feel like a weighty tragedy. A relationship with God gives meaning, supplies purpose, and provides direction to life. These are all things we desperately desire for our children. As Catholics, we have been catechized to trust in God. We are to use those things the Catholic Church offers such as prayer, the sacraments, and Holy Mass as the means to deepen our relationship with him and grow in likeness to Christ. The information in the previous chapters, however interesting and even insightful it may have been, would not be categorized as healing tools. The purpose of this chapter is to take a closer look at how our Catholic faith can assist us in our effort to help those who suffer from a poor body image.

Prayer

Prayer is an aspiration of the heart, it is a simple glance directed to heaven, it is a cry of gratitude and love in the midst of trail as well as joy; finally, it is something great, supernatural, which expands my soul and unites me to Jesus.

— Saint Thérèse of Lisieux

A friend of mine (then in the seminary, now a priest) said the single biggest impact on his vocation was his father. But his father never pushed or even encouraged his son or any of his other children to serve the Church by being a priest or nun. Rather, my friend told me that he had vivid memories of his teenage years, seeing his dad kneeling while saying the rosary. While he never mentioned that his dad asked him to join in, my friend *did* say that it was something that literally led him to become a priest. My friend was captivated as he observed his father in prayer. First and foremost, he saw that his father had faith that God would hear his prayer. He also observed his father's humility as he knelt and made his way through the rosary. And think of it— humility, to a large degree, seems to be a lost trait. I notice on Sundays that few people kneel to pray before Mass begins whereas it seemed to be the norm growing up. Another case of being an old soul, I guess.

But something that should never go out of style is teaching our children the basic tenets of prayer. And one of the critical aspects of prayer is to be honest when we struggle with things like a poor body image. Take comfort that Scripture tells us over and over again that consistent and specific prayer is key (cf., Phil 4:6-7; Matt 7:7). By providing the details of our hopes and intentions we acknowledge our weaknesses. This is directly tied to our humility, and humility leads us to a better, more meaningful relationship with God. A prayerful life of conversation with God solidifies that relationship. However, addressing vague concerns regarding our body image limits us in prayer, and limits us from laying hold on God's grace as well. A child's prayer should include asking for forgiveness (for inappropriately desiring the "perfect" body), giving thanks and praise (for the body we have), and petitioning God for spiritual, mental, or physical healing (e.g., for fortitude to avoid the issues and situations that trigger a negative view of our body).

To learn the most about a good prayer life, we should turn to Jesus. He taught his disciples the basic tenets of prayer (Our Father, Matt 6:9-13), to pray when distressed (Matt 26: 36-44), and to pray often (John 11:42-43). All are important when we seek healing.

I remember the nuns preparing us for first communion when I was in the second grade. They specifically addressed what to do after we receive the Eucharist. They instructed us to return to our pew, kneel, and pray. They encouraged us to pray in gratitude for what we have been given. We were instructed to give thanks for our brothers and sisters, parents, and even our favorite toy or our pet. The nuns also said that we should petition God for things that we think would make the world better such as stopping war (then the Vietnam era) or healing someone who is sick. Now as adults, we all know that those are pretty standard petitions, but as a seven-year-old I didn't. I am thankful for those nuns and Catholic schooling in general because that's when I first learned to pray. However, many parents feel that faith formation at the local parish or simply regular attendance at Mass will teach our children how to pray. While it's possible that some, even great prayer-based wisdom will be learned from a source other than the parent, it is not prudent to think this way in most cases. In other words, parents bear the primary responsibility to teach their children the art of a prayerful life.

You will probably have their attention best on such issues when they're young, so take advantage of this fact. Regularly encourage them to be honest with themselves and with God, and to include petitions designed to help them draw closer to our Lord. Specifically, gently instruct your kids to address prayer for the reasons just mentioned (variety of petitions and thanks and praise). Regularly passing along this teaching is one of the primary ways of developing a prayerful, faithful, and ultimately fulfilled child.

When it comes to body image, helping your son or daughter lead a life of acceptance and gratitude helps lead them to the peaceful state that we all desire for them. Expressing gratitude for our blessings, for life itself, and for a body to live that life in the world is how we begin to develop that peace. And consider this: What if we only got today what we thanked God for yesterday? What a scary question.

While prayer should not be governed by fear, pondering the above question could be a great motivator toward daily interaction with God. And by the way, what would be wrong with using it as a motivator? Either way, frequent reflection on the body as a gift—something especially needed on days when we're feeling down on our bodies—is perhaps the best way to combat the demons of body distortion.

Every day we make an important choice to fill our hearts with gratitude *or* be a complainer. It is difficult to always know how God works, but perhaps his greatest reward to those who are grateful is to bless them with more gratitude. Conversely, when we fail to recognize his gifts, and do not thank him for them, we fail to recognize God's love and deprive ourselves of the very graces he wills us to have. In fact, some of our most rudimentary actions allow us to draw closer to our Creator. Being able to kneel, fold our hands, and slightly bow our heads enable us to demonstrate that we are in prayer. It is obvious that even this most basic form of communicating with God is not possible without the body.

When we understand the greatness of God's gift, we begin to understand his divine plan—salvation. Since God formed us in the womb (Isa 44:24), there is a plan for each one of us. Being willed by God means that he wants us here, and our role is to determine why. It is through growing in this understanding that we become more thankful and come to fully realize what God asks of our bodies. Passing this along to our kids does not have to be daily task, but it should be taught consistently and in a somewhat plain manner.

I recently heard of the "Human Barbie," a woman whose fascination with the doll was so intense that she spent almost $1 million trying to be Barbie-perfect. Sadly, the level of peace in this gal must be tremendously low. This is an extreme example of someone who can't see anything clearly in life beyond seeking to perfect something that cannot be perfected. As referred to in chapter 4, seeking the look of Barbie, and Ken for that matter, is all too common. While not all plastic surgery is for cosmetic reasons, be assured that most of it is. And while we don't wish to dwell on stories like the "Human Barbie" (they do exist, by the way), perhaps we can use those sad examples to move us in a positive direction. Let's use them as an impetus to pray—for all who suffer from body distortion, and for safety from such burdens for us and for our children.

Praying for all who have similar struggles as well as for the thoughts that *we* have about being flawless can only help the cause of wellness and wholeness. As we pray on this, we do several things. First and foremost, we acknowledge the freedom-stripping power that searching for perfection brings. Second, we ask God to intervene in our thoughts and actions as well as those of others. And third, we directly display to God that we know the answer lies within him, his word, and the sacraments.

Saint Paul tells us to avoid being overly concerned or anxious in all matters, but to give thanks and praise to God. Through prayer, he promises us that *God's* peace will be upon us— the kind that (like God himself) transcends all understanding guards our hearts and minds in Christ (Phil 4:6,7). For those living in the anxiety-ridden world of body obsession, peace may seem out of reach. Their body obsession may be so powerful that they feel no one could possibly understand the depth of the problem. But God does. He hears the cry of those who suffer and wants to help us (Job

24:28). God is not the last hope—he is *the* hope. And children need to hear this Good News. Often.

Following are some age-appropriate suggestions to help you cultivate a grateful child through teaching on prayer.

Ages two to five: This is the age during which parents are most likely to pray with their children for the first time. Thus, this is the time to lay the groundwork in two vital areas. First, share the reasons for prayer (mentioned a few paragraphs ago). Second, teach and model gratitude—especially for our bodies. Help your children recognize that they are creations of God, with hands and feet that are specially designed for running, playing, and hugging mommy and daddy. I've seen (and read to my own kids) books that mention these things. Sadly, though, these truths are not commonly taught, nor are they emphasized as much as they could be.

Ages six to ten: Daily (or nightly) family prayer at this stage may fade, but many families still maintain group prayer periodically or once a week. When I was a kid, my family prayed together every Sunday night. By making weekly family prayer a priority, parents demonstrate not only how to pray but also the importance of prayer. Further, children start to develop a stronger body image identity at this age. This is when they may begin to wrestle with inadequacies that often stem from how others see them. Various prayers of gratitude will help temper any anxiety that starts to rear its head and will also cement the role that prayer plays in a fruitful life.

Ages eleven to eighteen: For a variety of reasons, when children reach adolescence and beyond family prayer becomes less common. In some cases, it simply stops. It could be easily argued, however, that these years are the most important years to pray with your children and help them make sense of things. These are the years that cause the most angst, especially for body-related issues. It's during these years that a certain level of "prayer maturity" should surface, but getting there usually requires some parental guidance. Not only is the conscience more formed, but also a deeper comprehension of the needs of others, as well as their own needs, has developed. Specifically, teens and pre-teens are starting to become aware of the role society plays in forming their body image. Two gifts of the Holy Spirit can assist them in their battle against the forces that create a poor body image—prudence and fortitude. Parents who communicate an understanding of what their children are going through not only display the needed empathy, but they can also close the loop by giving specifics on how regular and meaningful prayer eases body distortion.

Consider a prayer like this as part of your daily communication with God:

Lord, you know that I don't always like my body. And sometimes, I dislike it because it's not perfect. All of this worrying and complaining I do about my body is affecting the way I see and treat others, and it's keeping me from loving you the way I should. Lord, help me to accept the way you made me, and to turn my focus to serving others as you intended me to do. I love you for giving me a body that allows me to do so many things that are good, like hugging my friends and family members, playing my favorite sport, participating in the hobby I love, and reading a good book. I ask you God, to send your Holy Spirit upon me so I can fully appreciate this wonderful gift you have given me: my body. Amen

How and when God responds to prayer will always be a mystery, but we know that he does. We know that God answers prayer through our own experience, the testimonies of others, and Scripture. But perhaps the most influential way he answers and guides us is through our conscience. We were created to hear the voice of God, and that voice is constantly letting us know that he listens and that we can and *will* be healed. Our part is to consistently bring ourselves before God on bended knees and, with a humble tone, be direct in what we ask. Recall the fervor that Christ displayed in his agony at Gethsemane (Matt 26:36-39, 42, 44). Christ teaches us a great deal about prayer in those brief, intense moments. At his most vulnerable time, he turned to his Father—with perfect humility and all the passion he could muster—and he prayed.

In addition to petitioning, it's important to know that meaningful prayer extends to listening as well. When distorted thoughts of our bodies invade our minds, or on days when the urge to create a perfect body becomes powerful, it is then that God wants most to help us. Perhaps our prayer would be most effective when we ask direct questions such as, "God, how important is to you that I attain the perfect body?" Or, "God, would I be a better friend and son/daughter if I were less anxious about my body?" Or, "God, would my relationship with you be stronger if I could see my body as a gift and not as something to perfect?" Sincere and daily reflection on how God would answer these questions could open our hearts to the truth and put us on a road to true healing.

Confession

"In the life of the body a man is sometimes sick, and unless he takes medicine, he will die. Even so in the spiritual life a man is sick on account of sin. For that reason he needs medicine so that he may be restored to health; and this grace is bestowed in the Sacrament of Penance."

— Saint Thomas Aquinas

You might know that confession is also referred to as penance or reconciliation, but few know it as a sacrament of healing and the sacrament of conversion. Early in his papacy, Pope Francis provided "The Ten Reasons to go to Confession." Numbers six and seven, respectively, told us, "It is not a torture chamber where you'll be raked over the coals" and "Confession is an encounter with Jesus whose mercy motivates us to do better." These two comments directly relate to every sin we are likely to think of, and obsessing over body image is no exception. In one way or another, healing is what we need, and it is essential when we struggle with body distortion. Few afflictions, especially when extreme, are more paralyzing to everyday life. And sadly, anxiety over body image starts early in life for many.

Serious forms of body dissatisfaction, often at their worst when we are young, cast us into a world of persistent negative feelings. It's an existence of unaware self-absorption in which fear, pain, sadness, and various forms of self-hatred lead to a life of unhappiness and discontent. It's a life destined to break the hearts of watching parents. In such tough times, we have difficulty hearing God's voice, and we struggle with hearing and answering the needs of others. But as our current pope wisely observed, "When the door starts closing a bit because of our weakness and sins, confession reopens it."

God calls us to a life of holiness, and that includes the full acceptance of his gift to us—life itself as expressed through the body. Since man is sinful, the *full* redemption of the body will only be fulfilled at his own resurrection. Saint John Paul II encourages a life of virtue, growing purity of heart, and steady maturation toward perfection. By becoming more aware of our sinfulness, acknowledging our sins, and prostrating ourselves before the Lord, we grow in holiness.[1]

Although those who suffer from body distortion are (in a sense) victimized by it, we must also acknowledge that indulging in or perpetuating a poor body image can be sinful. It can have a damaging effect on us and those around us—even as we are blind to it.

---

[1] 12/9/81 TB.

First, we are sinning against others when we neglect to serve them because our thoughts, time, and money are absorbed by our obsession. Second, dressing immodestly in an attempt to attract others or to feel worthy indicates that we have lost the proper meaning of sex and the appropriate time to express it—privately within the context of marriage. The desire to feel sexy or to stir up lustful thoughts in others actually makes us an accessory to sin. Third, the constant dialogue with friends about the poor view we have of our bodies may generate similar feelings about themselves. But perhaps worse is no discussion at all with anyone. Lastly, we are sinning against God when we deny our body as a gift and instead adopt the dangerous notion, "If I have a nice body, there's reason to show it off." Where is the truth and dignity in that? It's insecurity or unawareness that leads to such behavior.

The sacrament of Confession gradually peels away the barriers between sin and virtue and allows us to be in full communion with God.[2] In this state, body distortion, selfishness, and pride fade away. *This* is the grace of God at work. And this is how we are healed. The healing that occurs from this sacrament brings us to a new understanding of God and his love. Love is what converts the heart into one capable of experiencing a new and joyful way of life.

Contemplate the very first quote from Christ in the Gospel of Mark: "The Kingdom of God is at hand. Repent, and believe in the gospel" (Mark 1:15). This is a call to conversion; and young people need to know God's mercy as soon as they comprehend this won-

---

[2] Saint John Paul II, in West, Christopher (2003). Theology of the Body Explained, Pauline Books, Boston, MA.

derful gift from God. Many people, especially Catholics, experience God's mercy in profound and memorable ways as a result of confession; so, wouldn't we want our kids to experience that, too? For the people who lived in the time of Christ, the gospel and their understanding of it was new. But we have heard it and need to be reminded of it so that we can remain in the way of Christ. Despite our level of education in the Catholic faith, we constantly need purification.[3] Seeking the sacrament of penance regularly can help us resist being enveloped by society's definition of the purpose of the body rather than God's. "If we confess our sins, he is faithful and just, and will forgive our sins and cleanse us from all unrighteousness" (1 John 1:9).

Here are some suggestions to help you cultivate a penitent, yet grateful child through confession.

Ages ten to fourteen: Many children of cradle Catholics first go to confession in the fourth grade. Although general discussions should take place about being appreciative of the body before age ten, the sacrament of confession is a perfect time for your children to become more conscious of the wonderful gift of their bodies. This age coincides with ramped-up discussions between friends about the body size, shape, etc., of others. It is also the time when they are growing in awareness of their own perceived flaws and where they stand in the world of attractiveness. Few (if any) books, talks, and parental encouragement can eliminate the angst of these years, but the sacrament of confession can encourage a heightened

---

[3] Catechism of the Catholic Church, No. 1428.

awareness of the issue. With guidance, something paralyzing can be converted into an experience of acceptance and thanks. Parents can gently call to the attention of their child a lack of gratitude about their body—especially if this attitude is combined with a noticeable and increasingly negative body image.

Ages fifteen to eighteen: As with prayer, regular participation in confession becomes less common during these years, sometimes because parents choose to "pick their battles" and focus on regular Mass attendance. But again, like prayer, the sacrament of penance can become such a tool of healing that children need to experience at this age as much as anytime in life. Later, teens tend toward notorious selfish behavior—just the kind of behavior that is fed by obsessive thoughts and a poor body image. Most priests aren't equipped to pointedly help someone wrestling with a negative body image. However, they can help strugglers put the issue into perspective by guiding them in the purging of sins and asking for forgiveness. And I encourage you as parents to share how your own experience in the confessional has led to a healthier and more meaningful life. Your role is to regularly lead them to penance and encourage a healthy confession; leave the rest to a good confessor and the Holy Spirit.

The Eucharist

"The Eucharist bathes the tormented soul in light and love. Then the soul appreciates these words, 'Come all you who are sick, I will restore your health.'"

- Saint Bernadette Soubirous

The greatest of all invitations is the one that Christ extended to us at the Last Supper. He offered us Holy Communion so that we could be in union with him.[4] By accepting his invitation, we can experience God's peace through separation from current sin and preservation from future sin.[5] Parents should teach their children that Holy Communion is powerful enough to wipe away the burden of a poor body image and even cure it. Simply put, parents must believe this before they can pass it on to their children.

As many of us know, the Eucharist means "giving thanks," and this includes gratitude for redemption, rescue from sin, and for creation. As to creation, we know that God not only made humans, but he also gave us "dominion" over what he created (Gen 1:26). Further, creation itself provides evidence that it was made for us with loving intent—a truly incredible gift in itself.[6] And as with all gifts, we should be thankful for it and let our thanks be stated – in our hearts and with our lips. This is why, as families, we should seek the Eucharist. Love of one another, ourselves, and God can

---

[4] Catechism of the Catholic Church, No. 1391.
[5] Catechism of the Catholic Church, No. 1393.
[6] 1/2/80, TB.

falter in the press of daily life, so we need this nourishment to die to the sin of body obsession and to live in a way that expresses our indebtedness to God for his great creation.[7]

In reference to regularly receiving communion, it reminds me of my old Hot Wheels play set (Yes, the toy cars). As a kid, my brothers and I owned several Hot Wheels cars as well as a small oval track for the cars to go around. One Christmas, we received a booster that attached to the track. This booster contained two battery-operated spinning wheels that propelled the cars around the entire track. Each lap, the cars would barely make it to the booster, only to be jetted around again once contact was made. The way I see it, the Eucharist can act like those rotating wheels, providing much-needed assistance when we need it most. Anxiety seems to be the norm for young people, especially concern about their bodies. What better "boost" can there be than to attend Mass and receive the Eucharist that is designed to reorient our attention and calm such issues?

When we deny ourselves the Eucharist, we are denying ourselves this unique presence of Christ and the help he holds out for the battles of everyday life. In those moments when our kids balk at Mass attendance, perhaps a gentle reminder of the healing power of Holy Communion would provide a change of heart. We want and need our Lord to remain in us, literally, to combat the barrage of TV ads, movies, music videos, and countless other distractions that can lead to a poor body image. Better yet, we need the power of Communion to help us *avoid* those triggers and turn more con-

---

[7] Catechism of the Catholic Church, No. 1394.

sistently toward those things which are good, noble, and pure. In fact, Christ gives his solemn promise that he will be with those who eat his flesh and blood (John 6:56). Passing this trust in God to our children will surely benefit those who seek him out. God knows the pain that body obsession brings. Encourage your children to bring that pain to him so he can do what he promises and heal our soul. This is why our response at the conclusion of the Eucharistic Prayer is so powerful: *Lord, I am not worthy that you enter under my roof, but only say the word and my soul shall be healed.* We are asking Christ to enter our body and heal our soul. Nothing is more powerful or more direct.

Here are some suggestions to help you cultivate a grateful child through the Eucharist.

Ages six to ten: The suggestions here are like the ones I gave for prayer. A basic discussion and reminder of what the Eucharist literally means (giving thanks) is a good place to begin. All children, whether they are in Faith Formation or attend Catholic school, need to be further catechized by their parents. There's nothing greater that a parent can do regarding the Catholic faith than to stress the importance, healing power, and sacredness of the Eucharist. Giving thanks after receiving communion will please God. And what father would not want to reward such a humble and grateful attitude?

Ages eleven to eighteen: As with prayer, a certain level of maturity is reached in the teenage years, allowing for an experience of the Eucharist's true power. Even inadequately catechized children sense the importance of communion as they see their parents kneeling and in prayer. No doubt, few things are more difficult than having meaningful conversations with some teens (e.g., regarding faith). But it is through such dialogue that the source and summit of our faith can make some real impact. Comments from a mom to a daughter such as, "I wish I had prayed more about lessening my anxieties about my body when I was your age," may be as calming as anything else we can say or do. Many teens confess that thoughts about their body and body image take up an inordinate amount of time and energy. What better healing tool could offer our children than to lead them to the One who takes anxiety away?

Mass

"In a world where there is so much noise, so much bewilderment, there is a need for silent adoration of Jesus concealed in the Host. Be assiduous in the prayer of adoration and teach it to the faithful. It is a source of comfort and light, particularly to those who are suffering."

- Pope Benedict XVI

"Protect us from all anxiety, as we wait in joyful hope for the coming of Our Savior, Jesus Christ." These are the words of the priest just prior to the Great Amen, the conclusion of the Eucharistic Prayer in Mass. It is a plea for God to pierce our hearts so that we can see that the bad times, although sometimes frequent, will pass and the peace of Christ will be with us.

Many young people who experience the stifling effects of an unhealthy body image need the peace that God has promised through his Son. At the center of the Catholic Church's life is the Mass.[8] It is here that we give thanks, ask for forgiveness, hear God's Word, and ask for strength from the Eucharist. While it is difficult for some children, even the ones who have received the sacraments at the traditional ages (i.e., Eucharist in the second grade, confession in the fourth grade, etc.), there are numerous teaching opportunities for parents to grasp as their child's curiosity and maturity develops. A complete understanding of the meaning of the Eucharist, comprehension of the lesson in a reading from the Old Testament, and knowledge of the history of the Mass are lifelong lessons. But all parents would serve their children well to simply focus on the Eucharist. It is the culmination of our Catholic faith and, ultimately, a display of the body's attempt to grow in communion with God. This is why the Catechism refers to the Eucharist as the source and summit of our faith.[9]

Since Christ is the full embodiment of God, this means that God can be seen, touched, and heard in the context of daily life. This principle is known as sacramentality, one of the defining characteristics of Catholicism. The Catholic Church regularly offers certain rituals, called sacraments, which make the presence of God tangible to us in a variety of ways. Sacraments mediate be-

---

[8] Catechism of the Catholic Church, No. 1343.
[9] Catechism of the Catholic Church, No. 1324.

tween God and his people, and these encounters are designed to deeply affect our lives. At the core of the sacraments is the Eucharist, and the Eucharist is at the core of the Mass.

We should encourage our kids to petition God through the Mass for forgiveness and healing of our body issues. Also, a deeper understanding of how we use our bodies will make us grow in appreciation for this gift. The Mass was instituted by Christ to allow our bodies to fully experience God through the use of our five senses—something most children don't think about and that many parents never think to convey. But the reality is that God has given us the ability to see, hear, smell, touch, and taste every aspect of the celebration. For instance, our encounter with Christ is enriched when we *see* the Host being raised, when we *hear* the Word of God, when we *smell* the incense, when we *touch* the Eucharist, and when we *taste* his Blood.

Without these senses—indeed, without our bodies—it would be very difficult to develop our relationship with God to the degree that he intended. Passing this along to children will serve them in two distinct ways. First, they will begin to view the body, in a general sense, as a holy creation. Second, they will be enlightened about the varied and powerful meanings of the Mass. And let's admit that if a parent can do the latter, that's one great accomplishment.

We should never let our children forget that God willed them to life. From the moment of conception, God desires that each of us know his Son in word and deed. Following the gospels points us in the direction of that gate of salvation.

The gospels are celebrated every time we go to Mass. Further, accepting the invitation to actively participate in every aspect of the Mass brings us closer to God. The body and soul work in tandem as our physical body allows participation and our soul reaps the benefit. This cooperation is neither coincidental nor simply a convenience. Without either a body or a soul, salvation would be impossible.

One of the recurring responsorial psalms at Mass is *"The Lord is my light and my salvation. In whom should I be afraid?"* (Ps 27). The beauty of this psalm is that it doesn't *really* pose a question, but rather makes a statement that is one of the basic tenets of Christianity. Conversely, a common question we hear during times of suggested or inevitable change is, "What are you afraid of?" Too often, fear governs our actions (or lack of action), especially when we are unaware that it is motivating us. Consider the role that fear plays in how we view our bodies (e.g., the fear generated by TV and magazine ads). Specifically, the formula for TV ads is cunning, yet simple: "If you don't use our product, you won't be attractive, sexy, masculine/feminine, etc.," or worse, "You won't be loveable." This fear tactic is used not only to sell a variety of weight-loss methods, but also to increase the level of dissatisfaction with a host of body parts that the ad-makers *know* the reader would like to change. Perhaps no single demographic is more vulnerable to these tactics than young people.

Advertising agencies successfully bombard us with a variety of effective strategies. Clever TV commercials, glossy magazine photos, imaginative internet ads and emails sent to personal accounts, and ads on the side of every social network site all chip away at our gratitude and contentment. The single most effective strategy they use is relentlessness. Because of the constant pressure, many people eventually concede and make an ill-advised purchase. Or just as bad, we become convinced that our perceived body flaws are as obvious to everyone else as they are to us. We believe that the product, promoted using the age-old tactic of fear, might lead us to happiness and contentment. We fear that we are doomed to fail in relationships, our jobs, etc., unless we use a specific product. But if that is true, then what is God's role in our lives? Is God something to contemplate at night only during our prayer time? Is God only to be worshipped on Sundays at Mass? Or does Psalm 27 have actual meaning in real daily life?

The Mass is deep and full of Christ's messages—many of which are direct—and one of the strongest messages addresses fear. During his passion, Christ experienced a great deal of fear himself. He knows this feeling well, and he is aware of the anxieties that our youth experience daily. It is interesting to note that products aimed at aging adults often capitalize on their fear of losing their youthful vibrant look. Since teenagers don't need youth, the ads aimed at them play on other fears, as mentioned. Part of the good news is that Christ views us with dignity and value regardless of our age, weight, shape, and relative degree of attractiveness. He wants us to experience a certain level of peace in our lives, and the Mass reminds us of that and encourages it. The following are part of the Mass, as either instituted or as an option:

"Grace to you and peace from God our Father and the Lord Jesus Christ" (Greeting);

"Glory to God in the highest, and on earth peace to people of good will" (Gloria);

"Be pleased to grant her (The Catholic Church) *peace"* (Eucharistic Prayer I);

"Deliver us, Lord, we pray, from every evil, graciously grant peace in our days" (The Doxology, following the Our Father);

"Peace I leave with you; my peace I give to you" (prior to the Sign of Peace);

"Now let's offer each other a Sign of Peace" (Sign of Peace); and

"Go in peace, glorifying the Lord by your life" (Concluding Rite).

The number of times that "peace" or "anxiety" is mentioned in the Mass indicates both the reality of it in our lives as well as how much God wants us to be free of those debilitating things. Christians, and most everyone else for that matter, want to live anxiety-free. We desire peace because we know that it brings a degree of happiness—many would say joy. However, most of us need help, even specific instruction, before we can experience the kind of harmony that results in joy-filled lives. This is the why the first of the theological virtues is faith. It becomes clear to each one of us when we are relatively young that life is difficult, unfair, and even mean. And sometimes we experience the meanness of life as a result of body image distortion.

Faith is meant to address those feelings and bring us back to a good and healthy place where Christ's words resonate. Faith is knowing with certainty that something awaits us after this life, that there is something more than this imperfect body. Trusting in the grace of the sacraments allows God's grace to penetrate our heart and mind. We are enabled to see that a perfect body is not part of God's plan. God's plan is for us to use the body in perfect ways.

Here are some suggestions to help you cultivate a grateful child and lessen body image-related anxiety through the Mass.

Ages two to five: Let's be honest, it's a victory to get *through* the Mass with kids this age. No one knows that better than Alecia and me—at this writing, our children are two, three, and four years old. Still, we try to communicate brief and periodic messages to them throughout the Mass. We may point to the crucifix and say, "There's Jesus; he loves you." Or when the Host is raised, we say, "That's Jesus." Or after the communion when everyone is kneeling and in prayer, we might say, "Let's be quiet so all of these people can keep praying to God." And if your parish is small enough to offer in-Mass baptisms, that a great time to say to your children, "You were baptized, too, and that's when you became a member of this church." This may well be the beginning of a sense of owner-ship for them. I think this age is a good time to develop in our chil-dren a basic reverence for church in general. And it can provide a fertile breeding ground for the sacraments they are about to re-ceive.

Ages six to ten: During these ages, the sacraments start to be-come a reality—especially the Eucharist since it is part of each Mass.

But even in the year prior to the conventional age of first receiving (ages six to seven), comments during Mass can include, "You'll be receiving the Host soon; it's a very special gift." And, "It'll be a great time to thank God for everything you've been given." It's a prime opportunity to encourage your kids to listen to the readings, the gospel, and the homily. You might latch onto one sentence or idea that was conveyed and apply it to their lives—perhaps something that relates to how God can help us in our struggles, including those involving body issues.

Ages eleven to eighteen: The meaning of, and appreciation and reverence for the Mass should continue to develop during these years. Attention spans and intellect develop also, giving parents opportunities for deeper conversation. Even on the short car ride to or from church, parents can elicit a point or two regarding how the Mass was "speaking" to their children. A question such as, "What was one point made during the homily that was memorable to you?" could lead to a teaching opportunity. Pointing out the number of times that "peace" is mentioned can help them comprehend the purpose of the Catholic faith. Parents who have worked to keep communication lines open may become aware of body distortion issues during these years. While directly addressing the struggle might be the most effective way to lessen their pain and anxiety, pointing them toward God through the Mass is another way to address our problem early enough to make an impact.

Accepting and fully practicing the faith can be challenging for an adult, and so can passing it on to our kids. But isn't the propagation of the faith one reason we had children? And we know that developing the faith of our children is the best thing we can do for them. The good news about "The Good News" is that it's worth pressing and pursuing. The efforts of parents to increase their child's faith lead directly to a greater understanding of why Christ left the sacraments to us. The sacraments are meant to fill us with God's grace, and that leads to emotional healing. But mom and dad must participate in the process. This part of the conversation is reminiscent of the story earlier in this chapter about the priest-to-be who observed his father at prayer. The son may have become a priest without his father's prayers and the prayerful example, but I'm sure none of us would bet on that. I know I wouldn't.

Here's another way to illustrate how prayer, the sacraments, and Holy Mass can help in the fight against body distortion: Let's say that the goal is to get over a big fence, and God is at the top of this fence reaching down with an outstretched arm. But we must climb up to meet him. While mysterious to an extent, poor body image does not develop by chance and rarely does it come out of nowhere. Perhaps the toughest thing to write in this book is that some parents, at least to some extent, may have to admit that they have inadvertently contributed to the frustration and pain of their child. I want to be gentle but direct here as I ask you to consider: Have you watched, or allowed your kids to watch racy TV programs or movies? Have you been too lenient with computer use, allowing your child to see inappropriate and potentially damaging images and videos on the internet? Have you purchased magazines that put all the focus on beauty and sexiness and very little on health? And you have sidestepped or not embraced the grace that our wonderful sacraments offer?

A virtuous life includes a certain degree of patience and fortitude. Building a household where praying and striving for the good in all things are priorities takes discipline and grace. Keep in mind that if life-long discipline and a close relationship with our Lord was the reward of receiving the Body of Christ just one or two times, or if all sin ceased after one confession, the offering of those sacraments would be rare. But it's not rare. In fact, we are asked to make Mass at least weekly and to receive the sacraments of confession regularly. In other words, our Catholic faith lived rightly is an everyday commitment. Saint Peter wrote: "Be clear-minded and alert. Your opponent, the devil, is prowling around like a roaring lion, looking for someone to devour" (1 Pet 5:8).

The "lion" in our case is the media's constant reminder about how we *should* look. This is how the media's strategy plays out: When ads appear featuring a perfect body, the image pounces on our brain, lingers, and then the inevitable occurs—your sons and daughters compare themselves to the image. Desire sets in, and when it is continually fed and fully developed, they begin to take the first steps to become more like the model in the ad. Few things are more powerful, and nothing seems to hold the soul prisoner more tightly than images that lessen the worth of the body that God has given us.

Volunteer

It's not coincidental that volunteer work is often directly associated with organized religion. And that's a good thing. Catholics only need to refer to James 2:14-26 where the apostle states that faith is dead without works, to justify volunteering. By no means the only way to demonstrate faith, volunteer work is concrete and can be a meaningful way to respond to God's call to service. Virtually every parish calls for unpaid workers in a variety of programs. Some needs are seasonal while others may be ongoing. Some are organized within the parish grounds, and others take place at nearby facilities.

A primary message of this book is that time spent fretting over bodily imperfections will leave little time and inclination to hear or do the word of God—I hope I've made that clear. On the other hand, let's consider some involvements by a teenager that might impact constant thoughts about being attractive, sexy, or thin. What about tending to the elderly in a retirement home, being a tutor in an immigrant community, serving dinner to the poor, or helping Down syndrome kids in a recreational setting? It is inevitable, at least to an extent, that people are more apt to put their anxieties into perspective when they *truly* experience others in need. Moreover, parents might want to seek volunteer situations with those who need physical assistance so the teens can fully develop an appreciation for their own healthy, fully functional body.

God intended that we live with full appreciation of our bodies, and he certainly does not want us to experience any of the anxiety and pain that accompanies the lack of bodily perfection. All pain is the result of the fall, and from that moment our need for God's grace has been acute. Due to God's gratuitous nature, we are blessed to have his grace constantly offered, but we must be willing and active participants in the process. The sacraments are the greatest gifts the Catholic Church can present. But they can be neglected or underappreciated, perhaps for the very reason that they are given so freely and are available to us every day. Because they are offered daily at no cost, we are called to receive the gifts they were designed to provide.

Through the sacraments, prayer, and unique experiences like volunteer work, God can calm the emotional storm caused by body obsession. Living with this struggle is like being tossed around in a violent storm that can seem to have the force of a hurricane. Let's give our children the shelter they need. Our shelter is our Catholic faith, and God is calling each of us to accept that faith.

Don't let the media or anything else determine your worth. Let God do that.

Chapter 6

Physical Activity:
Strive for Progress, Not for Perfection

Life and physical health are precious gifts entrusted to us by God.
We must take reasonable care of them, taking into account
the needs of others and the common good.

— Catechism of the Catholic Church (2288)

Everyone knows that exercise is good for everyone in the population. Young, old, pregnant, disabled, diabetic, obese, or hypertensive—all benefit from even just a few days of activity at low intensity levels. There's a *mountain* of data-driven literature out there that, if stacked, could probably reach the moon!

All of it confirms the value of a strong heart, healthy lungs, strong bones, and firm muscles. So, I'll spare you the additional rhetoric on "Why We Should Exercise." That said, *everyone* could benefit from some encouragement, and this includes our children. They especially need a dose of learned-behavior and that's where you come in.

So, let's take a look at some of the basics of increasing activity for our children.

Physical activity versus exercise

Many think of these terms as interchangeable, and they are, to a degree. But there is a difference, and it is magnified when applied to children. Exercise is what most of us think of when we use the term "workout." Exercise is a formal activity. It often has some specific parameters to it such as frequency, intensity, and duration of exercise. For instance, exercise is getting on the treadmill for thirty minutes, three times per week, at moderate intensity. Or it could be riding a stationary cycle, for forty-five minutes, four days a week, at low intensity. It may also include a resistance-training program of two sets of ten to twelve repetitions per muscle group. Because of the formality of this form of activity, it can be measured and improved.

And if it were a math equation, for many it would read something like this: Exercise = boring.

For that reason, most of us struggle with specific parameters, do a lot of clock-watching, don't really enjoy it (if we're *really* honest with ourselves), and often terminate our workout sessions within a couple of months—only to restart in the near future.

Physical activity is basically anything that causes our heart rate to rise, uses a few muscle groups, and improves overall fitness to some degree. This includes formal exercise but also includes less-formal pastimes like playing sports in the backyard, mowing the lawn, going for a walk after dinner, and taking the stairs rather than the elevator or escalator. The fact is, we struggle with any type of physical activity, formal or not. Consider this: In the 1970s and 80s, about two of every three students walked or biked to school.

Now it's one in eight. This tells us, for starters, that even one of the most common and fundamental activities for kids is now close to a rarity.

What we know is that if given a choice between exercise and physical activity, adults as well as kids would select physical activity. Of course, they would. Not only is it generally low intensity, but also there's a higher likelihood we'll have "fun" doing it. But the problem, whether we're talking about formal or informal activities is the same—just getting people to do it. Just like you, I have kids. And after a long day at the office, it's tough to agree to, say, two hours of hockey with the boy, or even jump rope with two wound-up little girls. I've been there. You're exhausted. Your mind is on a million different things. But we are not excused from that responsibility, are we?

So, we do it. And this not only pleases our kids, but guess who else it pleases? I'll drop a hint—the answer rhymes with God.

Just think how many times you've driven past a fast food restaurant with cars wrapped around the building waiting to pull to the drive-thru window and no one is inside the building ordering. Technology (including cars) has enabled us to take the easy route in too many situations. In addition to the drive-thru, consider delivery meals, delivery groceries, shopping online (not just at Christmas, but throughout the year), and Wii fitness.

Children, unless they learn healthy behavior early and often, can fall prey to the "technology effect." Traditional forms of movement are not just under-appreciated; they are virtually unknown to them! To increase the likelihood that our kids will enjoy and stick with being active, we need to strongly encourage them to engage in activities that avoid the parameters of traditional exercise. Now we can avoid such things as gauging intensity and monitoring the time. I know I really don't have to tell you this, but here are some ways to encourage your child to be active:

- ➢ Go to a park where climbing, jumping, and balance are required;
- ➢ Take the dog for a walk every day;
- ➢ Ride a bike to school, to a friend's house, or simply for the fun of it;
- ➢ Walk to do local errands (e.g., to the store, to deliver something to a neighbor);
- ➢ Disallow daytime TV watching, limit technology-based games, and encourage outside play with friends or siblings;
- ➢ Make purchases that encourage activity such as a trampoline, skateboard, a razor scooter, and the ever-favorite bike;
- ➢ Gauge interest in sports and purchase equipment so they can play regularly; and
- ➢ Play *with* them—doing anything. These occasions not only allow parents to assist their children as they learn a new skill, but also give their kids someone to play with and/or against. It also allows them to see you in a different light— parents having fun!

Think about how your children see you when you come home from work—necktie undone, briefcase in hand, and tired from the day. You just want to have some dinner and sit on the couch. In other words, the message delivered is, "Kids, life is over at thirty. Now it's just work, taxes, and death."

No, not really. Right?

I'd like to offer a suggestion: prepare yourself on the way home. Think of the fun you'll have for an hour before dinner is ready. Listen in your head to the sounds of children laughing and having fun. Try to recall what it was like when you were a kid. Remember how desperately you wanted your parents to spend time with you? Well, it hasn't changed. Your kids feel the same way. It's extremely important that parents live in front of their kids as people who practice what they preach. You want your kids to be active, right? We must remind ourselves that it works both ways.

Participation in Sports

Until this point, participation on sports teams has not been a part of the conversation, but not because I have anything against it. In fact, few people have played more team sports as a child (and even as an adult) than I have. Since grade school, I've been active. I played football, basketball, and baseball through high school. I went on to have a notable college baseball career, played rugby for several seasons (a history of broken bones is testimony), and played a year of professional baseball in Italy. To this day, I regularly cross train and engage in daily resistance training workouts. Okay, thanks for indulging me there. But my aim is not to boast, but to make a point. Even after fifty, we can remain active, alert, and a positive role model for our children.

Now drop and give me twenty!
Just kidding. (Well, kinda.)

But, there are a few things to consider when you sign-up your son or daughter for any kind of sports team. First, know that in most cases the traditional sports team's goal is not to increase physical activity, or to improve skills, but to win games. Sounds OK, right? Hold your horses. The win-at-all-cost mentality plays out in a hundred ways—most of them negative. Parents must grapple with a variety of situations like a coaching staff that berates their kid every time he or she does something mentally or physically wrong. They may also have to witness Junior getting no playing time because the coach fears losing ground if he or she plays anyone other than the starting players. Again, I've been there, and I get it. I'm as competitive as they come, and I want to win just like anybody else.

But here's what I'm getting at: activity-time in a traditional sport's practice is low and both teaching and bench time are high. The coach's objective is to teach plays, discuss strategies, and work on specific skills. For example, take a typical baseball practice. One person, often a coach, throws batting practice to one batter who gets a few swings while a couple of pitchers practice throwing on the side. Meanwhile, the others are scattered in the field awaiting a hit ball. Football, soccer, basketball, volleyball, and others each have their unique practice protocols and game dynamics, yet they all share the common trait of low activity-time. For this reason, participation in team sports should *not* be viewed as an alternative to weekly physical activity. Nor is it the solution to the well-documented inactivity and high body fat levels of today's child.

However, there is more to consider with sports participation. Some researchers have demonstrated that participants in team sports grapple with different body image-related issues than do those who simply exercise. These researchers investigated the difference in body image among high school girls who play sports, engage in formal exercise, and are sedentary. Further, they separated body image into two categories: aesthetic value and functional value. Aesthetic body image is an objectified view of the body. It focuses on those aesthetic qualities that tend to encourage girls to see their bodies from someone else's perspective. The aesthetic value has been associated with shame, heightened anxiety, and lower body satisfaction. Functional body image puts the focus on the physical capabilities or performance of a specific task such as playing a sport or working out.[1]

As most would anticipate, the research showed that athletes place a higher value on functional body image while those who exercise focus on aesthetic body image. This suggests that a young person's experience in sports is not identical to engaging in a formal exercise regimen. When the objective is success in relation to a

---

[1] Abbott, B., & Barber, B. (2011). Differences in functional and aesthetic body image between sedentary girls and girls involved in sports and physical activity: Does sport type make a difference?, Psychology of Sport and Exercise, 12, 333-342.

skill or outcome (e.g., winning the game) the participant tends to have a more positive view of the body. In other words, there is sense in which the athlete reflects on the body as a means to accomplish something. In sports settings, this is sometimes acknowledged as coaches and players say, "The game is bigger than you," and "There is no 'I' in team." Conversely, the researchers found that those who exercised placed more emphasis on the aesthetic qualities that others see (e.g., firmness of the arms, flat abs, shapely calf muscles, etc.). Such an emphasis may develop or confirm the kind of wrong thinking that sees genuine worth and self-esteem tied directly to physical beauty.

Moreover, seeing the body as a functional tool sets the stage for an understanding of the *Theology of the Body* when true understanding and appreciation of the body develops. Saint John Paul II is unmistakable in his words: "The body is a form of communication with God, with ourselves, and with one another."[2] The great gift of sport allows a unique form of communication. And the research referenced earlier showed that girls who play sports cultivate a positive form of communication with themselves. This in turn creates a better body image since thoughts center on the body's purpose and what it *can* do, rather than what it *can't* do. The following quote from JPII demonstrates that sport is not just a physical demand:

"Athletic activity, in fact, highlights not only man's valuable physical abilities, but also his intellectual and spiritual capaci-

---

[2] 2/4/81 TB.

ties. It is not just physical strength and muscular efficiency, but it also has a soul and must show its complete face. This is why a true athlete must not let himself be carried away by an obsession with physical perfection, or be enslaved by the rigid laws of production and consumption, or by purely utilitarian and hedonistic considerations."[3]

I have had countless male and female college students, often athletes, who have approached me over the years to inquire about achieving a perfect body. These young people, in almost every case, already looked good. Remember, they're *college students*.

But what they wanted was to look *really* good. They were probably casualties of aesthetic body image. On one occasion, a young woman brought in a fitness magazine and showed me photos of fitness-models she wanted to emulate. My comments were: "OK, I can give you a workout program and eating plan to get you to look like that, but your "fun meter" is probably going to drop off the charts. You can't eat sugar or fatty foods anymore, so that means no dessert or fast food; and you can't drink alcohol. Also, your workouts will need to be two to three hours per day of serious weight training and intense cardio sessions." As a result, her enthusiasm quickly waned, and the topic of conversation changed to something like the weather.

---

[3] Saint John Paul II, address to the international convention: "During the time of the Jubilee: The face and soul of sport", 9/28/00.

In these instances, the students seemed to realize that something was inherently unrealistic with their goals. They were like many young people today who are drawn to beauty and an appealing body shape but want it at little cost. But rarely do young people see the physical demands—not to mention the spiritual implications—that aspiring to such a great body can entail. A life dedicated to perfecting the body is an extreme one. The road to physical perfection is hilly, winding, bumpy—and ultimately endless. That's because just at the moment we gain a nicely proportioned and well-toned body, the first noticeable wrinkle will appear. What to do then? Buy wrinkle cream? Then apply and double apply, to get rid of it? Then what? Well, gray hairs begin to proliferate. So, we take care of that. Then a sunspot may appear in an inopportune place. Well, you get the idea.

This series of events takes place, in one way or another, to everyone. And I mean *everyone*. In spite of the all-consuming concerns of raising healthy children, attaining financial stability, and nurturing the family's faith, parents struggle with body image, also. When parents "age gracefully," it's because they make efforts to develop and maintain healthy habits. They display a certain balance that is not lost on their children. Young people inwardly yearn for this kind of stable environment. And all displays of healthy behavior by their parents, both mental and physical, will yield good fruit.

It's encouraging to know that most young people really desire a life based more on moderation. It's okay to include periodic rich, tasty foods in your diet and modest amounts of physical activity. We teach this to students at a relatively young age, and parents should encourage it. Many of today's parents of teenagers feel that their kids are underappreciated. The public generally views them as video game-playing slugs, ego-driven athletes and cheerleaders, or partiers. In fact, many teens are responsible, caring, and balanced individuals. They know that happiness doesn't come just from being physically appealing to everyone they meet. They have learned that the peace that God intends for us *not* reflected in today's magazine and internet photographs, TV shows, and racy movie scenes. Maybe some of us just got lucky to have kids like this. But let's give at least some credit to the parents who have provided this insight.

Activity other than sports and exercise

Other ways to increase physical activity include school recess, physical education (PE) class, and regular visits to the local park. Recess, often seen as just a necessary break for the teacher, has been shown to provide more activity time than a more stifling PE class. Plus, due to its informal nature, recess allows children to select from a variety of games, activities, and sports. This naturally leads to more involvement due to greater interest. Think about it: what would *you* rather play, a sport picked out for you, or one that you *actually* enjoy?

Although PE provides fewer opportunities for free play, by design it educates in numerous ways and encourages play beyond the gymnasium. And it can encourage healthy habits long after schooling stops. Like recess, local parks provide a setting for the kind of free play that allows children to prosper and creativity to develop.

Interestingly, PE, recess, and parks each has a local or state government component. That is, each may come to a vote in one way or another. I have known local school districts to vote on whether to eliminate recess, or whether to increase or decrease PE. I have also seen residents vote on measures to build or expand parks. It is good to note that signing a petition, casting a vote, or contacting a politician are additional ways in which we can encourage more healthy lifestyles and noticeable differences in our communities and schools.

The entire discussion of this chapter thus far directly relates back to body image in several ways. Let's recap:

First, it has been established that kids who play often don't deal with weight-issues.

Check.

This means they will have a better body image.

Check.

Most people see the inherent good in improving the health of a community.

Check again.

But since better health directly affects a child's body image, there's now one more reason to fight for any measure that increases activity time. Having your child engage in physical activity places the focus on something potentially wholesome and fruitful while diverting their attention away from the TV and other countless other forms of technology. Let's face it, physically speaking, allowing your kids to watch too much television can cause them to be sluggish and unalert. How could it not? If all they see are commercials for glucose-coated sugar-bomb cereals and mind-bending video games all day, what do think will happen? You know the old adage for computers, right? Junk in, junk out. Yeah, works for kids, too.

The already-stated disturbing data on television viewing habits for teens (which tends to include computer games as part of "TV watching"), twenty to thirty-five hours per week is alarming. Even at the low end, it means at least three hours daily. These are colossal numbers that should move anyone to make an effort to lessen this common form of leisure.

Every couple of weeks, my wife and I pile the kids in the car and meet another family from church at a local bagel shop. One time while driving home after meeting our friends for bagels, our four-year-old Clare said, "Daddy, they didn't say I was pretty." After stumbling over my words for a few seconds, I said, "Well, no sweetie, they didn't. But you *do* look pretty today. However, what God likes is when we do good things because he wants us to be pretty on the inside." If this seems contrived for the purpose of this book, let me assure you that it is not. In fact, it not only happened exactly this way, but I spent the next two or three minutes on the "pretty on-the-inside" theme until I felt she got the point. After all, what an ideal opportunity.

Until now, I've avoided mentioning that the goal of eating and exercise should be to look good. Frankly, there's nothing wrong with either looking good or being good-looking. Looking good is usually a combination of healthy habits, spending some time in front of the mirror, and tasteful clothing selection. But being good looking from conception is akin to being struck by lightning. How can you think you had anything to do with it and take credit? Instead, recognize the source of beauty and thank God for the blessing.

Looking good is an appropriate goal for healthy living. It does nothing to separate us from God. But looking good should not be *the* goal. In fact, one reason we should not really aspire to be more attractive is that it will naturally occur when we take care of ourselves. It's kind of like having a good vegetable garden. If you use rich soil, water regularly, and shovel in a pinch of love, you'll produce a fine crop. Now you may not produce the 400-pound pumpkin or seventeen-pound squash you see at the 4H fair, but you'll still have pretty good, healthy table food.

So, back to health. Less body fat, more toned muscles, increased energy, strong posture, and better circulation are all-natural outcomes of healthy habits—and all especially noticeable in the face. Sometimes, the only motivation we *really* need is to recognize that something is the right thing to do. And that's the case with eating right and exercise. A household mantra, reflecting a healthy way of living, will resonate in the minds of young people. The results will suppress thoughts of how others see us and elevate how God sees us. This, in turn, will have a healthy effect on how we see ourselves.

So, I know what you're thinking: I have a salad tonight with my family, and my kids won't need a shrink later on in life? Not quite, but you get the idea.

An exception to the principle of not thinking too much about how others see us is the natural appeal we want to have when it comes to relationships. Teaching right thinking and behavior about this is another of the many (and complex) responsibilities of parents. Adolescents and certainly teens naturally strive to be seen as attractive. So how do we, as parents, manage this raging river through a rocky gorge? My first suggestion is to never deny the power of physical attraction. Nothing will make a parent seem more clueless than that. Address and acknowledge its influence, but put it into perspective. That is, when talks about the body start, be sure to keep God's perspective as a part of the conversation. God is pleased when our intent is to glorify him, and taking care of the body is just one way we do that. A healthy, more attractive body is the result of good practices. The key to having conversations like this with children is to, for lack of a better word, prioritize. When entering into discussions with children about physical attractiveness, it's vital to delicately frame the conversation around the concept of the body being God's greatest gift. Taking care of our body is something God expects us to do. You might also stress that a natural outcome of taking care of our body contributes to making us "good catch." The earlier we use such dialogue with our children, and the more often in their lives we reinforce it, the more impact it will have.

A major theme of this book is that glossy, manipulated images and many other factors (discussed at length in chapter two) do not reflect reality. Aspiring to mimic these images cripples any chance at developing a healthy body image. Therefore, a topic that should be addressed, at least concerning health and fitness, is weight and the percentage of body fat. Magazines, entertainment shows, and daily conversations put all the emphasis on body weight and size and rarely on health and happiness. However, I say with some trepidation that there are valid reasons to watch our weight and body fat. I just don't want to add to the hysteria—I want to calm it. But here we go anyway.

It is a fact that teens and young adults, as well as the general population, can be anywhere on the spectrum of thin to morbidly obese and *still* suffer from body dissatisfaction. Many who suffer from body distortion are so thin and/or muscular that a dose of reality is desperately needed. For this reason, responsibly addressing the topic of weight and body fat is important.

For a given height, the body mass index (BMI) is proportional to weight, thus making it easy to calculate an appropriate size. While considered flawed for a few reasons (e.g., if listed as "overweight" BMI cannot distinguish if the weight is excess fat or excess muscle), BMI is accepted as a legitimate means to determine healthy body weight. And having your BMI measures is simple and comfortable since no touching occurs and the only information needed is height and weight (see BMI chart and ratings). A more precise and direct way to figure appropriate body composition is by testing the percentage of body fat. Skin calipers, body-fat analyzers (e.g., Bod Pod), and underwater weighing are the most popular and valid methods to determine body fat (see percent body fat chart). But as I've stated, it's unfortunate that many remain anxious over their bodies despite seeing that they are within the healthy ranges of BMI and body fat percentages. Above all else, we need to convey the non-existing relationship between body fat and dignity as human beings.

Look for a moment at some historical figures that we perceived as "overweight" but who still managed to prosper and serve others.

Excess body fat did not keep icons like Winston Churchill, Oprah Winfrey, and Santa Claus from earning respect and being effective in their jobs. And the list could go on. Most importantly, we are no less loved by God or any less dignified if we don't meet the BMI standards of the latest magazine model, bodybuilder, or pro athlete. That stated, there are practical reasons (e.g., health and daily productivity) to aspire to a healthy body weight. So, body mass index and percent body fat charts can be a gauge to motivate and assist the effort needed to change and adopt healthier habits. Here they are:

Body Mass Index Chart

(see next pages)

		Wgt. (lbs)							
Height (in)	Height	100	105	110	115	120	125	130	135
58	4'10"	21	22	23	24	25	26	27	28
59	4'11"	20	21	22	23	24	25	26	27
60	5'0"	20	21	21	22	23	24	25	26
61	5'1"	19	20	21	22	23	24	25	25
62	5'2"	18	19	20	21	22	23	24	25
63	5'3"	18	19	20	20	21	22	23	24
64	5'4"	17	18	19	20	21	21	22	23
65	5'5"	17	17	18	19	20	21	22	22
66	5'6"	16	17	18	19	19	20	21	22
67	5'7"	16	16	17	18	19	20	20	21
68	5'8"	15	16	17	18	18	19	20	21
69	5'9"	15	16	16	17	18	18	19	20
70	5'10"	14	15	16	17	17	18	19	19
71	5'11"	14	15	15	16	17	17	18	19
72	6'0"	14	14	15	16	16	17	18	18
73	6'1"	13	14	15	15	16	16	17	18
74	6'2"	13	13	14	15	15	16	17	17
75	6'3"	13	13	14	14	15	16	16	17
76	6'4"	12	13	13	14	15	15	16	16

195	190	185	180	175	170	165	160	155	150	145	140
41	40	39	38	37	36	35	34	32	31	30	29
39	38	37	36	35	34	33	32	31	30	29	28
38	37	36	35	34	33	32	31	30	29	28	27
37	36	35	34	33	32	31	30	29	28	27	27
36	35	34	33	32	31	30	29	28	27	27	26
35	34	33	32	31	30	29	28	28	27	26	25
34	33	32	31	30	29	28	28	27	26	25	24
33	32	31	30	29	28	28	27	26	25	24	23
32	31	30	29	28	27	27	26	25	24	23	23
31	30	29	28	27	27	26	25	24	24	23	22
30	29	28	27	27	26	25	24	24	23	22	21
29	28	27	27	26	25	24	24	23	22	21	21
28	27	27	26	25	24	24	23	22	22	21	20
27	27	26	25	24	24	23	22	22	21	20	20
27	26	25	24	24	23	22	22	21	20	20	19
26	25	24	24	23	22	22	21	20	20	19	19
25	24	24	23	23	22	21	21	20	19	19	18
24	24	23	23	22	21	21	20	19	19	18	18
24	23	23	22	21	21	20	20	19	18	18	17

255	250	245	240	235	230	225	220	215	210	205	200
53	52	51	50	49	48	47	46	45	44	43	42
52	51	50	49	48	47	46	45	44	43	41	40
50	49	48	47	46	45	44	43	42	41	40	39
48	47	46	45	44	44	43	42	41	40	39	38
47	46	45	44	43	42	41	40	39	38	38	37
45	44	43	43	42	41	40	39	38	37	36	36
44	43	42	41	40	40	39	38	37	36	35	34
43	42	41	40	39	38	38	37	36	35	34	33
41	40	40	39	38	37	36	36	35	34	33	32
40	39	38	38	37	36	35	35	34	33	32	31
39	38	37	37	36	35	34	34	33	32	31	30
38	37	36	36	35	34	33	33	32	31	30	30
37	36	35	35	34	33	32	32	31	30	29	29
36	35	34	34	33	32	31	31	30	29	29	28
35	34	33	33	32	31	31	30	29	29	28	27
34	33	32	32	31	30	30	29	28	28	27	26
33	32	32	31	30	30	29	28	28	27	26	26
32	31	31	30	29	29	28	28	27	26	26	25
31	30	30	29	29	28	27	27	26	26	25	24

275	270	265	260
58	57	56	54
56	55	54	53
54	53	52	51
52	51	50	49
50	49	49	48
49	48	47	46
	46	46	45
	45	44	43
	44	43	42
	42	42	41
	41	40	40
	40	39	38
	39	38	37
	38	37	36
	37	36	35
	36	35	34
	35	34	33
	34	33	33
	33	32	32

BMI Ranges:	
Underweight	< 20
Ideal	20-25
Overweight	25-30
Obese	> 30

Percent Body Fat Chart

Body Type	Female	Male
Excessively Lean	<10%	<5%
Lean	12-22%	6-15%
Normal	22-25%	15-18%
Above Average	25-29%	18-20%
Overfat	29-35%	20-25%
Clinically Obese	35+%	25+%

This is not the first attempt to place in perspective the relationship of healthy habits and God. Several books have been written that attempt to address these issues, such as "Does God Care How Much I Weigh?" and "Does God Care What I Eat?" The authors conclude, to no one's surprise, that God does indeed care about how we treat our bodies, and he expects that we will treat them with dignity. But that makes sense, doesn't it?

Several popes throughout history have been strong supporters of physical health, advocating sport and physical activity.[4] Popes Saint Pius XII (1939-1958) and Saint John Paul II both spoke and wrote extensively about the role that physical activity plays in society as well as the role that morality and moderation play in the life of the athlete. Not surprisingly, the Vatican under JPII, instituted The Office of Church and Sport that addresses expectations for the moral dimensions of life for athletes as well as those who oversee sport. Among its purposes, this new office for the laity directs the

---

[4] Catechism of the Catholic Church, No. 2288, 2289.

athlete to see all forms of exercise as means to develop the mind, soul, and body as God intended (more on this in Chapter 9). So clearly, the Catholic Church encourages the human person to be physically active, but always within the framework of the church's teaching.[5] In conclusion, we understand that being in good shape is good and even Godly, but does God really care how well an athlete does a touchdown dance? I doubt it.

It's obvious that we should be aware of any action that tends toward obsession or a negative view of the body, but we must also be careful when relying on others who might weigh in on what it means to be fit or attractive. Fitness "experts," beauticians, surgeons, and others may be guilty of promoting obsessive behavior themselves. Encouraging our children to regularly participate in physical activities will help them avoid the trap of body obsession. So, by now we get the picture: shut off the TV, toss the Xbox into the hall closet, kick the kids off the couch, and get outside.

Despite the general encouragement to lead a healthy lifestyle, keep in mind that even the strictest personal trainer allows a day or two off per week. Nor would a trainer frown on the *occasional* fast food meal or bowl of Neapolitan ice cream. However, just as with our sacramental and prayer life, healthy behaviors need to be modeled and practiced with regularity. This is the way healthy behaviors become healthy habits that lead to healthy benefits that remain. As we saw earlier, we must accept responsibility for reading and watching things that harm our body image. Likewise, we must

---

[5] See Robert Feeney's book "A Catholic Perspective: Physical Exercise and Sports," Ignatius Press, 1995.

also accept responsibility for excess body fat and poor fitness levels resulting from inactivity. Parents, particularly, must take responsibility. Despite any ambivalence that you (and I) have, body fat and body mass index need to be respected. Habitual bad eating and lack of physical activity generally leads to a high BMI, which in turn plays a direct role in poor body issues.[6] Conversely, the data correlating moderate and consistent exercise regimens[7] (and even one-bout sessions of light physical activity) with a positive body image have been consistent.[8]

When diet and exercise regimens become extreme in either direction, it is problematic. Alarms should sound when the desire to achieve a better body morphs into getting absolutely "ripped" or into a belief that thinner we are, the better our lives will be. On the other hand, a lack of effort to care for the body is just as troubling. Obsessing over the perfect body means neither do we have the time, nor do we care to meet the needs of others. Conversely, poor

[6] Weaver, A. & Byers, E. (2006). The relationships among body image, body mass index, exercise, and sexual functioning in heterosexual women, *Psychology of Women Quarterly, 30*, 333-339.

[7] Henry, R., Anshel, M. & Michael, T. (2006). Effects of aerobic and circuit training on fitness and body image among women, *Journal of Sport Behavior, 29*, 281-303; Hausenblas, H., & Fallon, E. (2002). Relationship among body image, exercise behavior and exercise dependence symptoms, *International Journal of Eating Disorders, 32*, 179-185.

[8] Scarpa, S., Nart, A., Gobbi, E. & Carraro, A. (2011). Does women's attitudinal state body image improve after one session of posture correction exercises?. *Social Behavior & Personality: An International Journal, 39*, 1045-1052; Sabiston, C. M., Pila, E., Vani, M., & Thogersen-Ntoumani, C. (2019). Body image, physical activity, and sport: A scoping review. *Psychology of Sport and Exercise, 42*, 48-57.

eating and exercise habits result in bad health and low energy levels that also have a negative impact on our ability and desire to help others. In short, we need to be healthy to serve as God has commanded.

Are these concepts relatively easy to understand? Is it difficult for many to eat healthy and exercise regularly? Is it difficult to turn away from the images that elevate the awareness of our body's imperfections? Yes, all three times. But that's the purpose of this book, and it relates to the reason for Christ's birth, death, and resurrection. The central purpose of this book is to draw attention to the relationship between the coming of Christ to us and the power to overcome the dangers associated with a distorted body image.

Being honest with ourselves, with those around us, and in the confessional is not easy. But being true to ourselves sets us on the road to lower anxiety and a closer relationship with God. Developing an obsession with our bodies is incongruent with and disrespectful of Saint JPII's central theme in *Theology of the Body*—that an appropriate use of the body is at the core of God's divine plan. The great pope set out to change the way we see our bodies. He makes it clear that our primary task in life is to experience the love of God and share the language of God's love with others. While this book doesn't have the power to heal body distortion, it can play a part in exposing the issue. And it can extend two of the most powerful healing tools that our faith has to offer: *Theology of the Body* and our wonderful sacraments.

Don't let the media or anything else determine your worth. Let God do that.

Chapter 7

Nutrition: Follow the "80/20" Rule

It is not the soul alone that should be healthy; if the mind is healthy in a healthy body, all will be healthy and much better prepared to give God greater service.

— Saint Ignatius

I once saw a cartoon with two little girls looking curiously at a scale. One girl said to the other, "Don't step on it, it'll make you cry." Like so many jokes, it's funny because it contains truth and is, well, *funny*. But it is no laughing matter to acknowledge that we are a nation of overweight people. Obesity numbers have never been this high. We're losing the "Battle of the Bulge," and the root of the issue can often be traced to health habits developed early in life.

As a result of the general preoccupation with health in our culture, few issues are more discussed and analyzed than nutrition. In fact, we might safely say that nutrition has become an obsession. Conversations regarding food cover everything from whether foods are good for you, portion size, mealtimes, and meal frequency to the benefits of eating upside down, underwater, in zero gravity, or at 3:16 in the morning. The proliferation of various diets is so much a part of our everyday life that even when the information varies slightly from one source to another, it sends us into a state of "dietary confusion." And to add to this confusion, only diet books currently outsell cookbooks. Hmmm. I'm sensing a bit of a nationwide dichotomy here. It's hard to blame consumers for being so leery when the number of "experts" steering us toward (or away from) a particular eating plan is so high that computer would have trouble keeping count.

I sincerely believe that some (even well-educated) people create new diets or put a twist on traditional diets because it's something different and therefore it sells. Why? Because people have become desperate. Common recommendations such as: eat several small meals daily, drink plenty of water, and glean around 50% of your calories from complex carbohydrates, are ignored or looked at with a jaded eye. But these suggestions have been around for decades. Yes, this *is* your father's diet. But the percentage of overweight and obese people keeps rising. Could it be that we mistakenly cling to the notion that whatever is new must be better than what we've been doing?

Probably.

But as a result, we question even the best eating plans and venture headlong into diets that are arbitrary, potentially unhealthy, or don't meet basic nutritional requirements. Some of us have even embraced diets that include hamburgers, chocolate cake, and pizza as staples. How does this happen? First, we see the plan presented with all the bells and whistles on a grand stage (e.g., popular morning shows). It may even include some pseudo-science, or it's being promoted by a razor-thin actress. Next, we ignore the sirens when they go off in our head—you know, the ones that signal fraud. At times like this, it is so important to stop and think. And if it is hard for us to discern the right thing to do, how difficult must it be for our kids once they start hearing these messages?

Just as with the previous chapter on physical activity, the purpose here is to encourage, educate, relate the basics of nutrition, and point our health-o-meters in the right direction. While this is not designed to be a book on nutrition, I feel compelled to bring some good, sound thinking to the world of eating, especially as it relates to body image. Parents who are conscientious in health matters are far more likely to raise healthy children. Beyond morality and faith, there's no other single issue confronting the family that's more important than teaching healthy nutrition. The literature on the impact of poor nutrition on health (including healthy body image) is vast. But the bottom line is and always will be this: we should aim for 80 percent of our meals and snacks to be healthy; and with the remaining 20 percent, we can take some liberty every couple of days. To clarify this point, here's my attempt to right this nutritional ship.

So, what should we feed our children?

This is not going to be about what we *shouldn't* feed our kids. Everyone knows that dessert, most fast food selections, soda, and highly processed foods such as hotdogs and many boxed products are not good choices. To be honest, my family doesn't avoid these foods altogether. But we do limit them, and all families should attempt the same goal. In fact, my wife and I have decided not to introduce soda to our kids since I believe it may be the single biggest contributor to obesity and many other diet-related conditions. We'll see if that sticks the day they walk into McDonalds with their teenage group of friends. I do know this though: my mother *never* allowed soda in our house and, as a result, I very rarely drink it. My point is: get 'em while they're young, my friends.

In the late 1990s, a true dietary revolution began. Within just a few years of one another, books and programs such as The Zone, Atkins Diet, and The South Beach Diet were introduced. They captivated our nation with a "protein is good and carbs are bad" approach. Since that time, it's hard to keep count of the number of similar books that have popped up. For a few years now, The Paleo Diet has led the pack.

Because I was a new professor around the time the original high-protein diet books became popular, I decided to look further into the phenomenon. I remember one that stated something like, "You've been told since the 1960s to follow The Food Pyramid eating plan: eat lots of grains, a moderate number of fruits and vegetables, and limited amounts of protein/meats, fats and sweets. But note the vast number of obese, diabetic and low-energy Americans." I became frustrated at this point, since the author failed to mention that most Americans were not following The Food Pyramid. So how could following its guidelines be blamed for low levels of overall health? When my frustration faded, I became impressed with the clever route the authors had taken. They continuously pointed out that The Food Pyramid was not working and pointed to people's waistlines and early death as their proof.

It was an ingenious strategy, something to rival Bill Gates' plan to get a P.C. into every home and hut in the world. And it was also a good way to sell a lot of books. They steered people away from the government's suggested nutritional plan by simultaneously inferring that traditional meals are outdated. They planted a seed, hoping to see it mature into some type of food euphoria in their readers. Eventually, they introduced the new plan: a high-protein/low carbohydrate diet that was unheard of prior to the year 2000. It quickly resonated with our "Neanderthal" mentality that encouraged us to believe we should consume as much meat as we could stomach. At the same time, these eating plans condemned many vegetables and just about all fruit. In other words, they gave us "permission" to adopt the very type of diet that was shunned by nutritional experts. However, one very good and necessary truth was pressed home in these programs: foods that cause blood sugar to suddenly rise (e.g., soda and most conventional desserts) have no nutritional value. They pointed out that these foods are harmful in the fight against obesity and many common conditions such as diabetes. And they were right.

Even though health professionals have long suggested that high-sugar foods are not good for us, it was the high-protein diet advocates who elevated this concept to an unprecedented level. Since then, various other movements have managed to keep it in the forefront. We know that high amounts of sugar cause the "insulin effect." When this happens, the body loses the ability to burn fat effectively, and thus focuses on using the sugar as energy (more on this in the next section). More recently, high-protein advocates have done a much better job of educating the public on the benefits of certain protein-rich foods (e.g., lentils and other beans, and soy products) and good-fat foods (e.g., avocados, nuts, and cooking oils such as canola and olive). Conversely, they did some damage in the process by lumping foods such as high-fiber breakfast cereal, and all bread, pasta, and rice in the "bad carbs" category. These food sources are still struggling to regain their reputation for being a healthy *part* of a sound nutritional plan, especially if you're active.

The Insulin Effect

After we eat a meal, blood sugar (aka blood glucose) rises. This is normal and, to an extent, good. Blood sugar is necessary for proper muscle, organ, and brain function. Blood sugar is also used as an energy source with the assistance of insulin, a hormone released from the pancreas. The problem arises when we eat meals or snacks that contain a lot of sugar (e.g., table sugar, honey, etc., also known as simple carbohydrates). They quickly convert to blood glucose, and the body struggles to use it all as energy. Pasta, rice, and bread (complex carbohydrates) can have this same impact on blood sugar but generally don't since they are often consumed with meals containing other nutrients that limit glucose levels.

Now, let's move to a major reason that high blood glucose levels are problematic. When we're at rest, about fifty percent of our energy comes from carbohydrates and the other fifty percent comes from fat stores. (Protein is primarily a cell-builder and can provide as little as five percent of our energy needs. Just ask anybody about energy levels during the first few weeks of the Atkins Diet). A few things can disrupt this fifty/fifty ratio (e.g., exercise or ingesting a lot of simple carbohydrates). Our focus, of course, is with the latter.

After eating high sugar meals, snacks, beverages, or desserts, our body focuses on the blood sugar and temporarily deemphasizes fat burning (depending upon how much sugar was consumed). So, rather than burning fifty percent of our calories from the fat candle, that number shifts downward to as little as twenty to thirty percent. A couple of major health issues arise because of this shift. Primarily, we burn less fat while the body handles the excess sugar. I liken the body's carb and fat burning to someone cooking a meal. Imagine the pasta water boiling over onto the stove (fat-burning) just when a small fire starts in the oven (sugar-burning). Both issues get the cook's attention, but the fire takes priority. When the body loses the ability to burn sugar effectively, it only spells trouble for parents trying to fight the fire of childhood obesity.

One or two high-sugar snacks every few days results in a few more calories of fat storage. But the calories in a few peanut butter nut bars or 24-ounce lattes everyday will eventually add up to additional *pounds* of fat, and obesity is a likely result. In addition to its impact on physical health, being overweight also leads to mental-related problems such as body distortion and poor self-esteem. These struggles often arise in children who are constantly being teased or thought of as too lazy and not talented enough for sports. For many of us, one look at our naked bodies sends our self-confidence plummeting. As a result, being active or playing sports is something we only do in our heads.

In addition to obesity, a diet that is high in sugar may lead to a now-common condition known as metabolic syndrome. This combination of ailments—increased blood pressure, high blood

sugar level, excess body fat around the waist, and abnormal choles-
terol levels—increases the risk of heart disease, stroke, and diabetes. Surprisingly, young people are not immune to this syndrome
since many have one or more of these conditions before they leave
their teens. As difficult as it is to imagine, some children are in dire
health straits before they can legally buy alcohol, tobacco, or even
vote. This begs a *troubling* question: America, what are we doing to
our kids?

Foods likely to raise blood sugar above normal levels

Fruit juice
Candy bars
Cake/brownies
Cookies
Pie
Ice cream
Sweet tea
Soda
High sugar breakfast cereal
Fruit bars
Pancakes/waffles with syrup

Again, keep in mind that the intensity of the insulin effect de-
pends not just on the sugary food, but *how much* of it is consumed
in a short period of time (e.g., ten to twenty minutes), as well as
what is eaten with it. A sip or two of soda has virtually no effect on
blood glucose, but thirty-two ounces of it in twenty minutes would.

Also note that none of this is absolute. There has always been some mystery to the impact of carbs and sugar on blood glucose. For reasons not quite understood, no two people handle sugar the same. Still, some things to think about that the next time you fill that half-gallon jug at the corner convenience store.

The U.S. Government's (and my) Recommendations on Nutrition

The United States government has made formal nutritional recommendations to the general public for about fifty years. It started in the 1960s but was elevated to an easy-to-read Food Pyramid in 1992, which was altered in 2005. Since 2011, the recommendations have been presented in the form of a plate, known as MyPlate. The first two pyramids were easy to understand but inherently flawed because they failed to make distinctions (e.g., differences in carbohydrate and fat choices). The current recommendations are much improved, especially since the whole concept is supported by a website. Where it could be difficult to make good dietary choices based solely upon a portion-based colored plate, the website explains suggestions and offers options.

Despite some obvious and necessary changes over the years, one basic suggestion from the government has remained constant: around one-half of our calories should come from carbohydrates (at least forty up to sixty percent), a moderate amount should come from fats (twenty-five to thirty percent), and, generally, the smallest portion should come from protein (ten to twenty-five percent). Numerous writers and health "experts" (including MDs) continue to plea for a re-thinking of the percentages reflected in the government's recommendations. However, it is rare for me to meet professionals in my field, including Registered Dietitians (RD) who would suggest anything other than minor fluctuations in these percentages. That is, virtually everyone who has professional training in nutrition (note that medical schools rarely require even one course) recommend that their clients, as well as their families and themselves, follow the basic information provided by MyPlate. Me included.

And, someone else.

Up to my late thirties, I knew a man who never read or even looked at a diet book. Yet his sensible eating habits still ring true for me to this day. He gardened, golfed, and participated in upland sports until he was in his mid-eighties. He remained thin and well-toned almost to the day he died. I remembered watching him eat. He consumed small, balanced portions at mealtimes, and *rarely* snacked on junk food. On his table were nuts and fruit and, oddly, an ashtray. He sometimes smoked a pipe and drank beer in moderation (neither of which I am condoning or endorsing here). But I believe it was his regular healthy, sensible eating choices that balanced his very occasional less healthy indulgences. He remained vibrant, athletic, and mentally keen his whole life. Who was this man? My grandfather. No one told him how to eat. He didn't refer to calorie cards, and he never saw an infomercial. He just lived and ate sensibly. Why? Because it just made sense.

So, while it's easy to get swayed by a beautiful actress making a cleverly worded pitch on TV, fancy words in an article, or an MD's recommendation in a book, beware. You just might be searching for something you *want* to hear rather than something you *need* to hear. We've all heard it said that if it sounds too good to be true, it probably is. Remember that the job of marketers is to sell their product, regardless of the truth of the claims or whether the product is actually good for you. And this especially goes for nutrition. You can get dizzy trying to keep up with an author's rationale for trying his or her new diet. Instead, why not imply use my grandfather's brand of common sense as you make choices for yourself and your children? Raw fruit is much better than a fruit bar, vegetables are always great choices, chicken and turkey are better choices than beef and pork, a bowl of low sugar and high fiber cereal or a couple of eggs is better than a stack of pancakes, and a glass of water is better than a glass of . . . well, just about anything else.

Furthermore, too many diet purveyors put the primary focus on *what* we eat. While this is significant, concentrating on how *much* we eat is even more important. If there were such a group as the "Nutrition Police," the first change they would make would be to ban "All You Can Eat" buffets. The age-old suggestion of eating five or six smaller meals each day is still sound. It forces the eater to manage portions by developing awareness. If I know that I will be eating again in two hours, I am less inclined to overeat now. Common sense. Thanks again, Gramps!

Here are some commonsense recommendations regarding meals and snacks:

Suggestions for Breakfast

— Oatmeal with raisins and walnuts
— Cereals that combine carbohydrates with moderate protein and a modest amount of fiber (e.g., three to eight grams per serving)
— Omelet or eggs, with or without your choice of meat and cheese
— Fiber-based bagel with cream cheese
— Note on breakfast: Try to combine carbs with protein, fat. and fiber. Carbs and fats take notably longer to digest thus will keep us full longer.

Suggestions for lunch

— Turkey/chicken/chicken salad or tuna fish sandwich, with lettuce and tomato; served with crackers and cheese, carrot sticks with hummus, piece of fruit
— Hearty soup (e.g., lentil, bean, split pea, chicken noodle) with a grilled cheese sandwich, piece of fruit
— Egg and cheese on a bagel, crackers, piece of fruit
— Yogurt, crackers and cheese, vegetables with ranch dressing, fruit
— Hearty salad

Suggestions for dinner

— Pasta with steamed broccoli and chicken, bread

— Rice, bean, and chicken burritos, with cheese, sour cream, and lettuce

— Grilled chicken breast, steamed green beans, pasta with Parmesan cheese

— Spaghetti with chicken or turkey sausage, salad, bread

— Broiled fish (e.g., salmon, haddock, tilapia), sweet potatoes, pasta or rice dish

— A "Big Salad": lettuce and plenty of other vegetables, along with hard boiled eggs, meat-protein, and cheese.

Note that many of the protein-rich foods in these meals exclude pork (e.g., sausage, bacon, ham, etc.), and beef (e.g., steak, hamburgers, roast beef, etc.), to emphasize that "white" meat and seafood are better choices. While periodic meals with these meats are okay, pork and beef tend to be much higher in saturated fat which increases the chance of heart disease more than turkey and chicken. This usually correlates to more calories as well. Also, as I offer these meal plans, my goal is to make general suggestions. Each can be altered according to finances, availability of food, and family preferences.

The internet is also a tool to help your family with nutrition in two different, distinct ways. First, there are thousands of recipes for every type of food. If you want 365 ways to serve chicken, it's there. If you want to know what vegetables go best with a certain fish, it's there. What's the best way to make pizza at home? That's there too. Next, consider using a free online tool known as Super Tracker at https://www.choosemyplate.gov. This software is designed to analyze anyone's food intake. It examines if you are within the general suggestions of caloric consumption, as well as appropriate balance of macronutrients (carbohydrates, fat, and protein) and micronutrients (vitamins and minerals). This program can be used to analyze daily, weekly, or monthly food intake. It's easy to use, and I can ensure you that you will find it helpful and insightful. Side note: I have been an instructor of a nutrition class for sport science students for fifteen years. My students consistently say that being required to use this very program to analyze their diets is one of the most effective and helpful assignments they have as undergraduates.

And now that I've put you in an information-based coma, let's take a story break.

One of my brothers was a fireman for the City of Detroit. He once told me that the two communal meals he shared with his fellow firefighters were among the highlights of his day. But the best part wasn't necessarily the eating of those meals; it was the preparation. They would play the radio, joke, and laugh while each man took to his assigned meal prep task. One guy would make the salad while the other fired-up the grill. Another would make the sides while another would set the table. It always sounded like so much fun to me (especially while I ate my cold sandwich in the faculty break room to Muzak's version of Michael Jackson's "Billy Jean"). So, adopt the firemen's attitude and try this at home. Make meal preparation fun and educational. Is it practical to do this every day at every meal? Probably not. But most days throw in as much joy and adventure as you can muster – in preparation and during the meal. This not only helps build a strong family unit, but it can make healthy eating virtually painless. And, as we've learned from our reading, eating healthy can lead to a better quality of life, better self-esteem, robust health, improved body image, and so on.

Okay, back to the book.

As parents, we must also acknowledge the impact that our own eating has on our children. Just as with exercise, there's an abundance of nutrition-based information to sift through. What and when should I eat? What are the best foods to increase energy and boost metabolism? The basics of healthy eating, however, can be easily understood in the new MyPlate. The "plate" seen below is simplified and easy to understand. Grains and vegetables should dominate most meals while fruit and dairy products, to a lesser degree, should also be a part of your daily intake of calories. Beans, eggs, and meats can also be a substantial portion of some meals. Note that high (especially saturated) fat and high sugar-based products such as desserts and sweetened beverages are suggested in minimal amounts. In fact, using MyPlate in concert with Super-Tracker to analyze daily meals can provide valuable insight about healthy eating.

Despite the general encouragement to lead a healthy lifestyle, keep in mind that even I would allow an occasional slice or two (or three) of pizza. Neither would I raise an eyebrow to the occasional wedge of apple or pumpkin pie (homemade, of course). However, just as with our sacramental and prayer life, healthy behaviors need to be *regularly* practiced if we expect to reap any clear benefit. And just as we acknowledged the ways we assimilate media offerings and other things that harm our body image, we must also admit that excess body fat and poor fitness levels did not magically appear. Healing begins when we concede that we have made bad choices along the way—choices that directly lead to poor health-related conditions. Habitual bad eating and lack of physical activity generally lead to a high BMI and play a direct part in poor body issues.

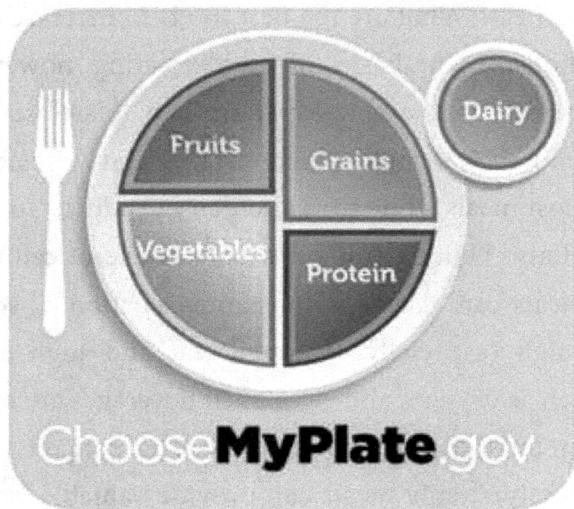

For more details on the food pyramid see http://www.mypyramid.gov/

Ten Tips for Better Nutrition

1. **The inside of your refrigerator should be colorful.** The most naturally colored foods are fruits and vegetables. Granted, some fruits and vegetables take time to prepare, but they are good for you for a reason. One of the most confusing (and frustrating) suggestions made by some nutrition "experts" is to limit your intake of fruit and many vegetables since they may raise blood sugar. But

raising blood sugar is not problematic in itself since it occurs after we eat just about anything. Also, some have hinted that eating a piece of fruit is no better than having a piece of cake.

Don't you believe it.

Cake is far denser in calories, has limited vitamins and minerals, contains saturated fat, and has no fiber. Fruit, on the other hand, contains fiber, is rich in certain vitamins and minerals, and provides some water. Overall, fruit and vegetables offer a variety of vitamins and minerals, and often contain at least a modest amount of fiber. Fiber helps to manage hunger and plays a major role in healthy eating. So, anyone who raises a caution flag over fruits and vegetables should be looked upon with suspicion. By their rich and vibrant colors alone, these foods can grab the interest of children. Three things are key: begin offering them to your children early in life (remember, healthy habits begin when we are young), offer them regularly, and offer a variety.

Recall when you were a kid and rolled that Brussels sprout around on your plate until it turned into an icefall. *You* didn't like all foods, fruits and vegetables included. So don't get discouraged when your kids make a funny face when you present some of these foods to them. Just try again later. And finally, there's been a lot of chatter about which fruits and vegetables are best: fresh, canned, or cooked. I say, who cares? Just get your kids to eat them.

2. **Offer salad or some type of vegetable at every dinner.** Although our daughter Clare has eaten salads since she was about two and a half, this may be more appropriate advice for parents of

teenagers. While everyone doesn't love vegetables, it is usually more appealing when it is part of a meal (rather than *the* meal). Also, due to the perception that salad and vegetables prep generally takes a lot of time, it'll more likely be consumed if it is to their liking. People may argue that certain salad dressings or vegetables cooked in butter or oil are best avoided – and for good reason, but the most important issue is the vegetables. To add taste and a few more nutrients to a salad for instance, replace iceberg lettuce with romaine or butter lettuce and throw in a few other vegetables such as broccoli, cucumber, carrots, and tomatoes. You can even add chicken, cheese, nuts, and hard-boiled eggs. Offer a couple dressings and you might get more interest than you think. Regarding vegetables, seek out new ways of preparation. An example: I disliked, rather, hated Brussel sprouts as a kid. But now Alecia bakes them with a touch of balsamic vinegar and a touch of maple syrup, and I literally ask her to make them weekly. Our children like them too.

3. **Offer snacks that contain more than carbs.** Many snacks for kids are often carbohydrate-based, and there's nothing wrong with that. Good examples include applesauce, pretzels, crackers, and fruit. However, to avoid blood-sugar spikes that are followed by a sudden dip, consider snacks like yogurt and peanut butter that combine carbs with fats and protein. Other examples of good combinations include crackers with cheese, nuts with raisins or Craisins, breakfast cereal with milk, veggies with hummus, and a small bagel with cream cheese. Contrary to popular belief, snacks are not a bad idea. *Bad* snacks are a bad idea since some parents disguise

dessert as snacks. In addition to allowing you to diversify the nutrients in your child's diet, snacks offer healthy options to condition them to eat smaller portions.

4. Make dessert special. Undeniably, our country has an addiction to sugar. Sugar addiction is not a condition to take lightly as there is a growing amount of literature that strengthens this theory.[1] We cannot, nor should we, avoid sugar completely. We must accept that almost every food contains some sugar or other sweeteners. However, it's vital that we see dessert for what it is: a poor nutritional choice that should be limited in both amount and frequency. But note: the word I chose was "limited" and not "omitted." To avoid dessert all together would be unnecessary as well as unrealistic. On the other hand, we must respect the dense calorie-content of most desserts and the overall damage it can do to one's health over decades. While there is no guarantee that limiting your dessert intake will transfer to similar behaviors in your kids later in life, you will do them a great service by demonstrating that dessert should be just a once per week, on special occasions, and holiday treats. Once again, this came from my own mother who only pre-

---

[1] Onaolapo, A. Y., Onaolapo, O. J., & Olowe, O. A. (2020). An overview of addiction to sugar. *Dietary Sugar, Salt and Fat in Human Health*, 195-216; Johnson, P. & Kenny, P. (2010). Dopamine D2 Receptors in Addiction-Like Reward Dysfunction and Compulsive Eating in Obese Rats. *Nature Neuroscience, 13*(5): 635-641; Volkow, N., Wang, G., Fowler, J. & Telang, F. (2008). Overlapping neuronal circuits in addiction and obesity: evidence of systems pathology. *Philosophical Transactions of the Royal Society Biological Sciences, 363*(1507), 3191-3200.

pared dessert on Sundays. Many addictions set their roots early in life. For this reason, in the realm of nutrition, parents are responsible for establishing good eating habits that will transfer to adulthood. Making a commitment to a few important changes, even small ones, will serve your children well in the future.

5. **Water should be the house beverage.** The irony of the bottled water craze that began in the mid-1990s was that it coincided with the phrase, "Obesity is now an epidemic." While obesity has been a concern since the early 1900s, today it affects two-thirds of adults, and the concern has climbed with each rise in the percentage. I believe that the single biggest factor in this epidemic is not choosing water on a daily basis. Soda (diet or regular), sweet tea, coffee beverages (like white chocolate mochas and Frappuccinos), and sports drinks are nutrient weak and disrupt the metabolism to some degree (see "insulin effect" earlier).

Bottled, tap, filtered, or any non-caloric water are good choices. All other beverages (with the exceptions of unsweetened tea or coffee, and flavored water) should be looked at from same angle as dessert. Like dessert, these beverages fail to meet any basic nutritional guidelines, may add to the problem of the "insulin effect," and are huge contributors to the nation's obesity problem. Consider this: one pound of fat is equivalent to 3,500 calories. Therefore, to gain one pound of extra weight in a month, we would have to consume 3,500 more calories than we expend.

But weight gain is far subtler than this. Let's say a man is maintaining his weight for one month; that is, he is neither consuming more nor fewer calories than he is expending. However, if he adds one regular soda per day to his diet for the next month, this adds up to 4,200 additional calories he is ingesting. If his level of activity stays the same, that means he will gain slightly more than one pound. In a year, he will have gained twelve pounds. That means his ten-year high school reunion rolls around, and Stevie the Stud has become Peter who is pleasantly plump.

6. **Diversify proteins.** Many families tend to confine protein-based foods to beef and chicken. Others branch out and get regular servings of protein through pork and turkey and, to a smaller extent, seek out cheese and milk. While meat is at the top of the list for foods high in protein, consider offering any type of fish or seafood, eggs, yogurt, a variety of nuts, beans, and soy products. Since our family enjoys eggs in a variety of ways, just about every two weeks we have "breakfast for dinner" where we serve scrambled eggs mixed with chicken and cheese as the main course. We prepare toast and some type of vegetable to go with it so we're covering our nutritional bases. Teaching moderation is still key, but it's just as important to introduce balance and variety.

7. **Introduce fiber early in life and regularly serve foods high in it.** The high-fiber craze is relatively new on the nutritional scene, but it may be the best revolution in the past twenty years. The general suggestion for adults is to consume twenty-five to thirty-five grams of fiber per day. For our youth, it's just below that. In either case, meeting that guideline is no easy task, so it's no surprise that our nation is way behind in our attempt to meet this goal. Data

shows that we only consume ten to fifteen grams per day. Thus, a wise parent will make a concerted effort to introduce high-fiber foods early and offer them daily.

Fiber has gained a great deal of exposure and for good reason. First, fiber slows the absorption rate of food, including sugar-based foods, and thus helps avoid blood glucose spikes. Next, it's been suggested that fiber is good for colon health, which is important since colon cancer is increasingly common in both adult men and women. But even beyond these specific health-specific properties, the overriding reason for increasing fiber intake is that it reflects a good, healthy, balanced diet. That is, if we consume the correct amount of fiber, we're sure to be eating right. The good news is food manufacturers have gotten the memo. Everyday products are now higher in fiber than they used to be. This includes bread, pasta, chips and crackers, tortillas, and numerous breakfast cereals. In addition, most vegetables and fruit naturally contain fiber. Lastly, keep in mind that the terms "multi-grain," "stone-ground," "100 percent whole wheat," "seven-grain," and "cracked wheat" are increasingly common but may not be as good as they sound. Check the amount of fiber grams.

Furthermore, like most good habits, developing a fiber-rich diet takes work and regular attention. It won't just happen, and I won't suggest it's easy. High fiber foods need to be sought out so you will need to become accustomed to reading labels and doing other forms of basic nutritional homework. Try to avoid the "this can wait till they're older" attitude, especially when it comes to nutrition. Your efforts will pay off because it's a victory even if the changes your children makes are small. You are doing your entire family a great service by introducing a variety of good foods at the youngest age possible. And just remember: just keep dancing.

8. **Make gradual changes and progress slowly.** Regarding exercise, I once heard someone say, "Your goal is not to be the best, but to be better than yesterday." I believe the same is true for nutritional plans. A common mistake among new health professionals is making drastic changes to their clients' eating habits. Even though each suggestion may be warranted, too many changes are often overwhelming and, ultimately, unrealistic. In fact, a seasoned professional would create scenarios that allow for a series of successes with small changes, as well as provide strategies for each desired change. Change is not easy, and children are just as resistant to it as adults, although often for different reasons.

Still, here are two specific examples to help you increase the success rate of nutritional changes. Let's use cutting out soda as the first example. I've already noted that high-sugar, low nutritional value products like soda could (and should) be omitted from the diet. But the reality is many that people, young and old, enjoy soda and balk at the idea of omitting it altogether. Why not limit the intake by allowing your children to enjoy it only when the family eats out? Or perhaps you might allow soda just on Friday and Saturday night family meals. Maybe they can look forward to having soda for special occasions when Mom buys it at the store with other special items. Either way, know that this author, exercise physiologist, professor of nutrition, father of five, and all-around great guy is convinced that he can't devote enough time to the ills of drinking soda on a regular basis. So, I encourage you to make every effort to limit soda consumption and, dare I say, eventually cut it out altogether.

For the second example, let's go back to incorporating vegetables into every evening meal. Remember to ask your children which vegetables they prefer and offer a couple of options to go with them (hummus or salad dressing). Preparing them every night, even if it's simple, will create a routine that can pay off in a big way.

9. **Go out to eat and feel good about it.** Many parents see eating out as the "cheat-meal" of the week, but it really shouldn't be that way. Even if going out to eat means going to a fast food restaurant, you can accomplish three important goals. First, you can set a limit on what they consume. Once you arrive, look at the menu and provide choices: "Ok kids, you can have X, Y, or Z." Furthermore, you can insist that the beverage of the meal is water, at least some of the time. Putting limits on food and beverage choices will help you control the calories and the type of food they eat and will also model your new moderation mantra. Second, you are setting a precedent for each time you go out. Going to a restaurant can still be special, but you convey that the good eating habits you've established in the home are not just for home; they're for life. This is not to say that ordering pizza and having soda or going to an all-you-can-eat buffet is off limits, but such experiences should be the exception (twenty percent) and not the rule (eighty percent). Finally (and importantly in another respect), going out to eat will demonstrate how "normal" you are and how ordinary and easy healthy

eating can be. Everyone wants to be normal, especially kids. Just like dessert, going out to eat is a treat. And it can still be special without being rare.

10. **Set an example.** I purposely left this for the final suggestion. Most, if not all, of the previous nine tips lose much of their meaning if parents fail to demonstrate good, or at least moderate, nutritional habits. I recall seeing the movie *The Outsiders* when I was younger. There's a scene where an older guy, smoking in the hospital, is telling some teenagers not to smoke. One kid says, "but you smoke." And the man answers, "Yeah, but I'm older than you." But being older does not give you a hall pass for bad behavior. In fact, the older we get, the more aware of our choices we should become. Telling your kids to avoid soda, French fries, and brownies while you are consuming those very foods will have little impact. On the other hand, you will *not* be able to keep your children from eating all "bad" foods, nor should you. Mothers who have a positive body image make better choices for themselves as well for as their children.[2] But the opposite is true as well. This confirms that efforts by parents to control their own eating habits and engage in behaviors that assist in maintaining or losing weight (such as exercise) pay off in the health of their children.

I hope that these ten tips made a lot of sense to you, but I know that change can be intimidating. Changing our behavior is difficult

---

[2] Contento, I., Basch, C., & Zybert, P. (2003). Body image, weight, and food choices in Latina women and their young children. *Journal of Nutrition Behavior, 35,* 236-248.

to do and easy to sidestep. However, my primary goal in this chapter and the previous chapter on exercise has been to convey the relationship between healthy living and a positive body image. And I hope I have done it in a way that is, if you'll pardon the pun, easily digested. The benefits are worth it. In addition to an improved body image, the results from a healthy lifestyle include increased creative energy, more productivity, and better self-efficacy or the confidence to accomplish more. Parents don't want to instill these characteristics in their children? Still, the intimidation factor looms large. So, my suggestion is to choose one or two health-related changes and commit to just those. If you feel a dietitian, personal trainer, or wellness coach might help, I encourage you to contact one. But whether you make changes on your own, or enlist the help of others, you will find the rewards far outstrip and outlast the effort.

It's pretty hard to imagine anyone would disagree that God asks us to take care of this precious gift that is our body. If we make efforts to help our kids avoid images that feed body distortion, that's only meeting God halfway. An analogy from the world of nutrition would be limiting our efforts to avoiding *bad* foods. But we know that good eating means just that—to prepare and eat the *good* foods that energize our bodies while improving overall health.

Don't let the media or anything else determine your worth. Let God do that.

And avoid overeating. And soda.

Chapter 8

Myths and other Non-Truths about Body Image

Save me, LORD, from lying lips and from deceitful tongues.

— Psalm 120:2

In their 2002 book on body image, Cash and Pruzinsky began by pointing out that body image is a basic characteristic of being male and female, and it can have significant implications on physical and psychological health.[1] While that is certainly true, it is an incomplete truth as body image can impact our spiritual life as well. Anything that affects our physical and emotional health threatens our relationship with God and thus deserves attention. Hence this book. Moreover, just as with nutrition and exercise, I have found that misconceptions hover over body image like a condor over his prey. For that reason, I am dedicating these next few pages to dispelling some of the most common myths.

Myth #1: Only fit and lean people have a positive body image

Body image is one of the most perplexing and complicated concepts known to psychologists, sociologists, and health professionals. In particular, body image varies and morphs with multiple

---

[1] Cash, T.F. and Pruzinsky, T., (Eds). (2002). Body image: a handbook of theory, research, and clinical practice. New York: The Guilford Press.

factors and characteristics of the person. And body size is a predictor but not an absolute. To put this in perspective, think of the happiest person you know—maybe it's the jolly, heavyset gentleman you see at the market on Saturday afternoons, or your devil-may-care mechanic whose trim waistline went out with the Reagan administration. Then think of the frustrated souls who forever seem unhappy inside their perfectly trim bodies. An ideal weight, perky breasts, or perfect legs don't always equate to satisfaction in life. Some folks couldn't care less about the relative condition of their body. But for some men, the desire for less body fat, more muscle has been progressively more evident in the past three decades—even to the point of possible eating disorders. And for a century or more women have felt the pressure (from others or themselves) to acquire and maintain a perfect body.[2]

That said, desiring a more ideal body suggests some level of body dissatisfaction. Perhaps we just want to look good at the beach, or for our spouses; motives can be hard to pin down. However, in both adolescents and adults lower Body Mass Index (BMI;

---

[2] Pope, H. G., Phillips, K. A., & Olivardia, R. (2000). The Adonis Complex: The secret crisis of male body obsession. New York: The Free Press; Grogan, S. (2021). Body image: understanding body dissatisfaction in men, women and children, London/New York, Routledge; Cohen, R., Newton-John, T., & Slater, A. (2017). The relationship between Facebook and Instagram appearance-focused activities and body image concerns in young women. *Body image, 23,* 183-187; McCabe, M.P., & McGreevy, S. J. (2011). Role of media and peers on body change strategies among adult men: Is body size important? *European Eating Disorders Review, 19,* 438-446.

see chapter six) strongly correlates with better body satisfaction.[3] In other words, most people who have an appropriate weight— especially if it was acquired through healthy means like more exercise and better nutrition—are likely to have a more positive view of themselves. But earning a level of fitness and meeting a weight-related goal are only two of the things that may define a person's body image. Here are a couple of other examples.

Age. While people along the age continuum struggle with a poor body image, most research shows that those concerns diminish as we get older. Ironically, the twenty-year-old who exercises regularly and looks great in a bathing suit often has far more anxiety about his or her body than the sixty-year-old whose skimpy bathing suit days are a distant memory. Thankfully, as we mature, moments of pettiness and extreme self-consciousness are usually much less frequent.

Gender. While we've already established that females are far more likely to have some form of body distortion than males, both sexes are susceptible. And though too deep a dive for these pages,

---

[3] Duncan, M., Al-Nakeeb, Y., Nevill, A., &, Jones, M. (2006). Body dissatisfaction, body fat and physical activity in British children. *International Journal of Pediatric Obesity, 1*, 89-95; Ricciardelli, L., McCabe, M., Lillis, J., & Thomas, K. (2006). A longitudinal investigation of the development of weight and muscle concerns among preadolescent boys. *Journal of Youth and Adolescence, 2*, 177-187; Penkal, J., & Kurdeck, L. (2007). Gender and race differences in young adults' body dissatisfaction. *Personality and Individual Differences, 43*, 2270-2281; Watkins, J., Christie, C., & Chally, P. (2008). Relationship between body image and body mass index in college men. *Journal of American College Health, 57*, 95-100.

nationality, country of origin, and the societal norms of the culture in which we live play roles as well. I've tried to make it clear that while there are acts and experiences that alter body image for better or worse, there is no specific formula to predict or determine these things. Think of the human mind as one giant Rubik's Cube of thought and emotions. When you see it that way, it is easier to accept the moving complexity of body image issues.

Myth #2: Only attractive people have a good body image

This is a common myth for many reasons. For one thing, select media outlets are particularly good at promoting or strongly implying a robust relationship between physical attractiveness and happiness. Moreover, they're also pretty good at trying to show that being pretty or handsome correlates with confidence and a positive body image. As I've labored to illustrate, this can be accomplished with a single photo. Clever people in those ad agencies, huh? They have managed to convince many who suffer from body distortion that a minor flaw in their face (e.g., big ears, crooked teeth, balding, etc.,) means that no one could possibly view them as attractive. And this is the case even though they may objectively be considered good-looking. On this point, consider the following from the book, *The Broken Mirror: Understanding and Treating Body Dysmorphic Disorder*:

> One important and consistent finding by body-image researchers – and in clearly relevant to BDD [Body Dysmorphic Disorder] – is that this is only a weak association between subjective

body image and measures of objective attractiveness. The view from the "inside" (self-perception of physical appearance) doesn't match that from the "outside" (social perception of physical appearance) very well. In statistical terms, the two views of physical appearance typically share less than 10% variance. As [prolific body image researcher] Cash has stated, beauty is no guarantee of a favorable body image, nor is homeliness a decree for a negative body image.[4]

This common mismatch is a central aspect of BDD; people with BDD view their appearance – particularly their defective body area – very differently than others do. In addition, I've found that there's no association between the occurrence of BDD and actual overall attractiveness; BDD occurs in people of varying overall attractiveness, some of whom are very attractive. Further, I've found no association between the actual appearance of the perceived defect per se and severity of BDD symptoms – in other words, severity of BDD symptoms is just as great in those with no defect whatsoever as in those present (although slight) defect, just as in the rest of the population "insider" and "outsider" views clearly differ in BDD.

So, let's slice that into a more digestible piece of information: Cindy Crawford has a mole on her face. Does she care? Probably not. In fact, she turned it into a mark of beauty. Put the same mole

---

[4] Phillips, K. (1986). *The Broken Mirror: Understanding and Treating Body Dysmorphic Disorder.* New York: Oxford University Press.

on the face of someone who suffers from low self-image, and you have BDD.

Myth #3: Everyone with a poor body image has an eating disorder

Eating disorders such as bulimia and anorexia exist in about ten percent of females and about one percent of males, while as much as seventy percent of females and thirty-three percent of males experience some degree of a poor body image. So, it's possible to assume some type of relationship but, because the statistics don't match up, it is not a strong one. The National Eating Disorder Association suggests that eating disorders are too complex an issue to label simply one matter as the cause (e.g., poor body image), but it's safe to assume that simply not liking the way we look is one of the many roots of eating disorders. While a general dislike of the body is unproductive and potentially harmful, a poor body image has a range of effects. Periodic thoughts of being unattractive, the desire to exercise more, obsessive thoughts and actions (e.g., eating disorders or excessive cosmetic surgeries) are all numbered among the results of a poor body image. Before we move on too quickly, I'd like you to think about this: A friend of mine once dated a young woman who suffered from bulimia. In fact, her case became so severe that she eventually needed to have her front teeth replaced. You didn't miss-read that. The acid in her vomit actually caused her teeth to deteriorate to the point that she needed a new set of front choppers by the time she was twenty-five. By our American standards, she wasn't a "heavy" girl; so, weight had little to do with her problem. My friend later discovered that the young woman had suffered a traumatic childhood. As a result, her pain was manifested in an eating disorder. So, while it would be easy to label all people who suffer from eating disorders as weight-obsessed misfits, this isn't always the case.

Myth #4: African Americans and other minorities do not suffer from body distortion

A poor body image respects no boundaries of nationality. Among men and women of every nationality in the United States, there is a certain percentage that struggle with body issues. It's interesting to note that the research does show some correlation between ethnicity and body image (e.g., whites struggle more than blacks). However, it is the issue of how closely minorities relate to their ethnicity that determines the level of body satisfaction. For example, African American females who identified strongly with their ethnicity tended to have a better body image than did those who identified more with white culture in which thinness is considered ideal.[5]

---

[5] Coker, E., & Abraham, S. (2014). Body weight dissatisfaction: A comparison of women with and without eating disorders. *Eating Behaviors. 15*(3), 453-459; Oney, C., Cole, E., & Sellers, R. (2011). Racial identity and gender as moderators of the relationship between body image and self-esteem for African Americans. *Sex Roles, 65,* 619–631; Hesse-Biber, S., Livingston, S., Ramirez, D., Barko, E. B., & Johnson, A. L. (2010). Racial identity and body image among Black female college students attending predominantly White colleges. *Sex Roles, 63,* 697–711.

Blacks are often encouraged by family and other members of their communities to embrace curviness and to be confident in their body type. This, in part, explains why they may be more likely to have little or no body distortion. On the other hand, picture a black-tie affair at a country club. There you might see a thin, mature white woman gently take the wrist of a young debutante and discreetly remind her, "We don't get fat around here." Studies bear out that the white female is the demographic that includes the largest percentage of people with a poor body image. It would be easy to deduce that whites suffer the greatest body image problems since whites make up such a large percentage of the images seen on TV, movies, and the internet. Yet everyone can be affected by this issue simply because "thinness" is pervasive in so many social and media circles. Therefore, it's clear that parents of children of every ethnicity should be aware of the many contributors to the issue of body dissatisfaction.

Myth #5: The media is the only cause of a poor body issue

It would be negligent to place the blame for a poor body image solely on TV, magazines, and social media, but they could claim (along with the other causes discussed in chapter two) a healthy portion of that pie. One study is particularly worth noting. Researchers set out to determine body satisfaction levels in Taiwanese heterosexual men as compared to their United States counterparts. The results showed that the Taiwanese men displayed significantly less body dissatisfaction than the men in the United States. Upon investigation, it was found that advertisements aimed at males in

Taiwan magazines featured far fewer undressed men than did similar magazines for men in the United States. Those in the U.S. not only regularly contained ads featuring men in various states of undress, but also the models were typically more muscled than the average male.[6] This study underscores the validity of the Social Comparison Theory, which suggests that the more images we see (in this case, well-defined male models), the more likely we are to unfavorably compare ourselves to those images. And to be clear, multitudes of other studies have shown similar results.

The purpose of chapter two in this book was to demonstrate the depth and breadth of the body image issue. Parents who want to raise healthy, happy children simply must consider and come to terms with the information provided in this book and beyond. At the same time, we must respect the complexity of the human mind and acknowledge that it's impossible to pinpoint any one reason for the body image problems. Likewise, it's futile to try to determine the impact that this will have on our children. Just about anything that we may believe to be part of the problem probably is. The bottom line here is to trust your instincts. You know your children; you carried them to term, bathed them, fed them, and would recognize their cry from that of a thousand other babies. Now it's time to consider what you know about the triggers that impact them. Remember that there is not just one demon (collec-

---

[6] Yang, C., Gray, P., & Pope, G. (2005). Male body image in Taiwan versus the West: Yanggang Zhiqi meets the Adonis Complex. *American Journal of Psychiatry. 162*, 263-269.

tively, the media), but there are plenty of demons out there and there's more at play here than you might initially think.

Myth #6: The media only affects girls and women

The opening chapters of this book are devoted to the fact that this issue can afflict every person—male, female, young, and old. It is true that young females are more likely to have body image concerns, but we must recognize that anyone can develop a distorted view of his or her body. Many stories focus on females and their struggles with the impact of the media, but the media has done plenty of damage to the body image of males as well.[7]

In addition, two books from the same authors are worthwhile in the quest to arm ourselves with helpful information. One is titled *The Adonis Complex: The Secret Crisis of Male Body Obsession* (2000); the other is titled *The Adonis Complex: How to Identify, Treat, and Prevent Body Obsession in Men and Boys* (2002). While dated, they still convincingly demonstrate that males struggle with this issue more than most think and offer practical ways to combat male body distortion. In fact, the first Adonis Complex book is a

---

[7] Tiggemann, M. & Anderberg, I. (2020). Muscles and bare chests on Instagram: The effect of Influencers' fashion and fitspiration images on men's body image, Body Image, 35, 237-244; Warren, C., & Rios, R. (2013). The relationships among acculturation, acculturative stress, endorsement of Western media, social comparison, and body image in Hispanic male college Students. *Psychology of Men & Masculinity,*14, 192-201; Kerkez, F. (2013). Perception of ideal and healthy body image among preschool children. *International Journal of Academic Research, 5,* 114-119.

compelling read and the unofficial favorite of those who have en-rolled in my body image class. As touched upon in chapter four, the "traditional male" is not as commonly represented today as masculine and competent. Due in part to magazine ads and mov-ies, physicality receives more emphasis. Muscularity and a low per-centage of body fat are held up as the measure of a real man. Just look at today's ads that exploit fireman, cowboys, and construction workers. Only a hat identifies their occupation—the emphasis is on sweaty pecs and defined abs. So, now we men must be brave, smart, hardworking, *and* look good in a Speedo?

Myth #7: All who have a poor body image suffered from some type of trauma

Body image is influenced by many factors, only a few of which are traumatic. There is, however, a correlation between poor body image and sexual abuse and other disturbing experiences.[8] When a child begins to display characteristics of a poor body image, par-ents need to be attentive, inquisitive, and ready to engage in wise conversation. The issue may go deeper than a simple dislike of his

---

[8] Sack, M., Baroske-Leiner, K., & Lahman, C. (2010). Association of nonsexual and sexual traumatizations with body image and psychoso-matic symptoms in psychosomatic outpatients. *General Hospital Psychia-try, 32,* 315-320; Hajiyousef, H., Dehestani, M., & Darvish Molla, M. (2022). The Mediating Role of Emotion Regulation Difficulties in the Relationship between Abuse Experiences and Body Image Dissatisfaction among Adolescent Girls. *Journal of Applied Psychological Research, 13*(1), 327-344.

or her body. Thankfully, the increasing success of early detection of emotional or physical trauma is certain to lessen the impact of body distortion and a host of other issues.

Myth #8: People with a negative body image look in the mirror and only see "fat"

Although seeing fat where little or no fat exists may be the case for some, not all who struggle with a poor body image have such extremely distorted views of their bodies. On the other hand, it must be said that too much body fat is a very real issue that often goes beyond the nuisance stage. In the most severe eating disorders, such as anorexia and bulimia, there's a "hatred" of the body combined with an intense fear of weight gain. But otherwise, a poor body image manifests itself in a variety of ways. It is often intensified when situations of comparison occur—such as being the "negative" center of attention, or internalizing images seen on TV, in magazines, or on the internet. For centuries, parents have felt it necessary to chastise their daughters for immodest dress. Today, many parents are feeling the need to increase the pressure toward modesty due to the surrounding and powerful messages encouraging teens otherwise. As a result, parents are often labeled as strict, old-fashioned, and insensitive (whereas, we all know that the parent is actually being insightful, protective, and wise).

The motive of parents in these situations is simply to teach and encourage their daughters to embrace modesty and retain a certain level of dignity. This is a noble and important goal when raising wholesome children. One of the purposes of this book is to encourage parents to examine the role they can play in helping their children see the ways they may cause others to see themselves and their bodies in a negative light. For instance, consider the adolescent and teenage dance groups—the attire is often far from modest. Too many parents errantly think that these dance groups are innocent or that they are "just another extracurricular activity." But a wise observer will see that they often lead the participants to become competitive, extremely self-conscious, or both—sometimes even before the age of puberty. Sometimes, a poor body image can be magnified by attire. One study about cheerleaders reported that those who wore the most revealing uniforms experienced the most body dissatisfaction.[9] But that makes sense, doesn't it?

Unless the dance attire is modest (e.g., Irish Dancing), some parents I know have not allowed their children to engage in most forms of this activity and for good reason. Wouldn't you agree that this could be considered a way of protecting your child? Since involvement in some pursuits has been shown to have a greater risk of negative impact on your child's body image, steering your daughters towards more wholesome pursuits is not only wise but also kind. Helping them make better choices could save them countless years of drama, pain, and frustration. And consider this: How do you tell your teen to "cover up" later on when you let her "expose" as an adolescent in dance class? Since our oldest is only

---

[9] Torres-Mcgehee, T., Monsma, E., Dompier, T., & Washburn, S. (2012). Eating disorder risk and the role of clothing in collegiate cheerleaders' body images. *Journal of Athletic Training, 47,* 541-548.

five, we're far from the teen years, but I can imagine how hard it must be to reverse such things after setting such a precedent.

9. Myth #9: Body image issues arise when diet and exercise programs fail

Mark Twain once said, "Giving up smoking is the easiest thing in the world. I know because I've done it thousands of times." Twain teaches us an obvious truth in his inimitable style: behavior change is difficult; many who try to make a change encounter failure, and many fail multiple times. Every day, thousands of people in America start a diet or exercise program. And every day, many fail at that attempt. So, it's important to note that issues with body image aren't created when diet and exercise regimens fail. Rather, failure results in other emotional issues such as self-efficacy (the feeling that something can be accomplished), anger, frustration, and regret.

I once heard a tale of a young man's wife who decided that she was going to lose weight. As she put it, she wanted to have her "bikini body" back. The husband, to encourage her, offered her a cash incentive: one hundred dollars for each pound lost. If she were to hit her goal of losing thirty pounds, this would mean an extra three grand in her pocket. Now, it may seem crass, even rude, for a husband to offer his wife money to lose weight. But let's look at the spirit in which the offer was intended. The young man loved his wife dearly and didn't think she needed to lose even one pound. But he saw that she was determined, and understood the difficulty ahead for her, and figured a nice reward would help her along. So, she began a morning exercise routine that started off with three sessions a week. That diminished to once a week. Ultimately, it stalled at only a few times a month.

She didn't lose a pound.

So, Mark Twain was right, wasn't he? No matter what the proposed incentive, behavior change is challenging. Consider the 1983 hit movie *Easy Money*. For Rodney Dangerfield's character to inherit his mother-in-law's enormous fortune, he must quit smoking, drinking, gambling, and eating poorly. The hilarity (or sadness) of the film is to watch Monty Capuletti as he struggles with this dilemma: get rich, but cut out all the fun in life. Why is this funny? Well, to be honest, it really isn't. Remember, all comedies are tragedies turned humorous. But it's an all-too familiar situation for millions of Americans who are struggling to end one addiction or another. Now, most of us are not going to be offered wealth (or even three thousand dollars) to lose weight and become fit, secure, conscientious, and pious individuals. However, even when faced with the promise of a better lifestyle, better health, and better outlook, some of us would rather not give up our vices. Or maybe we simply don't have the tools to defeat them.

The key is to select strategies such as goal setting, social support, and reinforcement that increase the chance of success. Further, improving health through better nutritional habits and more physical activity has shown to improve body image, so any attempt should be considered noble as well as pleasing to God.

Wisdom (gained in part through language such as the *Theology of the Body*), a sincere prayer life, and receiving the sacraments regularly can combine to mount a potent defense against a powerful opponent. A sound nutritional plan and habitual exercise are not only inherently good, but simply make good sense in the overall picture. Since behavior change for most people is very difficult, it may be prudent to focus on just one or two changes (improving prayer life, attending Mass more often, or starting an exercise regimen, etc.) rather than multiple ones. In that way we can inch our way toward an improved body image and less anxiety.

10. Myth #10: Body image can't be changed

It is indeed possible to change body image; if it weren't, I would not have written this book. But to do so we need to see that God is the best and most powerful way and means. Consider the language of Saint John Paul II's *Theology of the Body* where he calls the human person "embodied spirituality." In other words, we are not bodies with souls, but rather we are souls with bodies. And we are asked to reflect what is in our heart and soul through everyday actions of the body. What troubles many young (and older) people is the disconnect between our spiritual life and everyday actions, our thoughts and our words. The most basic morals and ethics of society break down when we neglect to see the relationship between the physical body and the soul. That is, we often claim to be "faithful" people yet use our bodies in ways that offend God. Now, I'm not talking about living a sinless life—that's not possible. But I am saying that we must realize that not only are we unable to separate our spiritual side from our physical side, but combining the two is the very intention of God.

Early Church Father Saint Irenaeus was one of the first to elaborate on this concept. He defended the body against detractors who considered all flesh evil, and he explained its purpose. Saint Irenaeus taught that because the body is made in the image of God, and the soul has adopted the Spirit of the Father, we can legitimately work toward becoming the perfect human being. This is why we should strive for a harmonious relationship between our soul and our body. Irenaeus went on to say that living only for the body and its needs jeopardizes eternal life. But original sin can be overcome by accepting Christ so that we can be redeemed. In summary, too many desires—many of which require the physical body to carry out the act—create a separation between us and God.

Listening to and believing what secular society says about the body's purpose is often in direct conflict with what God has revealed. To clarify, a mature understanding of the body and its purpose as seen through the eyes of God can transform lives. And an improved body image is one fruit of that transformation. In *Theology of the Body*, our former pope has done a great service to those who struggle with body image. He clarifies the reason we are embodied. He has brought a certain language to the faithful so that we can better understand the body's purpose and has shaped this language so that we can clearly see the body as God's greatest gift. Hearing and embracing this language can be empowering and life changing. Saint John Paul II's words are part of the freedom that scripture says comes when we embrace the Truth (John 8:32). Body distortion issues can cause so much anxiety and frustration that all other matters, important or not, become secondary. Freedom from those consuming issues allows us to live the life that God intends for us: to use our bodies in ways that glorify him.

Don't let the media or anything else determine your worth. Let God do that.

Chapter 9

This Quote's for You

The body is not for immorality, but for the Lord, and the Lord is for the body.

1 Corinthians 6:13

One of the wonderful benefits of being a Christian is the availability of (and trust in) the written word of God. After all, words are sometimes all mortals have for guidance. For Catholics though, it goes beyond Scripture, which I argue is one of the beauties of being a member of this great faith. The saints and popes, for instance, have left volumes of wise words in their writings on a variety of topics. Their wisdom is potent and continually able to uplift and guide the faithful they most need it. In addition, the writings of our current and former popes are designed with the same intent. They are available to guide us in our everyday experiences—which leads to the purpose of this chapter. I have collected here some select quotes from a variety of sources that directly apply to body image and other topics such as sport and exercise. After each quote I provide, I'll offer some interpretation and also explain how parents can assimilate the information in their efforts to improve or maintain their child's body image.

1. *I praise you because I am fearfully and wonderfully made; your works are wonderful, I know that full well* (Ps 139:14).

This is a fairly well-known Bible verse from Psalm 139, familiar to many through its use in support of the pro-life movement. While it is indeed a powerful and pointed statement against abortion, it is also a general statement regarding God's greatest gift – the human person. It is interesting how the most amazing things can come to be taken for granted. Smartphones are a good example. What a fascinating technology we hold in the palm of our hands! Yet, what we first received with awe, we now commonly take for granted. Automobiles are another example. They've been around now for over a century, plenty long enough for us to become accustomed to them. Perhaps even more than computers and phones, they're considered commonplace and unremarkable despite being incredible pieces of machinery. Isn't it true that we are far more frustrated when our cars fail than impressed when they don't? Ah, humans.

Once, during a non-required faculty assembly, a biology professor gave a presentation on "The Beauty of Biology." With the assistance of slides, most of them of microscopic organisms, the professor provided some in-depth insight and interesting facts about the world of biology. It was a good presentation. He made several good points and achieved his goal of raising our awareness and level of gratitude for the world around us, and well, *in* us. We are fearfully and wonderfully made, indeed.

I appreciated the information so much that I decided to follow-up that presentation with one on "The Beauty of the Human

Body." As with cars, our tendency is to become frustrated and feel victimized when our bodies fail us. But, hey, shouldn't we spend a little time each day sending a shout-out to the God who made us, thanking him for this wonderful apparatus? Many Catholic colleges require a few philosophy and theology courses, right? Wouldn't it make sense if those same schools also required an Anatomy & Physiology course to develop a greater appreciation for the complex network of the human frame? Sure, it would. So, let's start a movement!

From the time our children are three to four years old, periodic comments about the wonders of the body can help them appreciate God's wonderful gift. How a cut heals, the fact that our heart beats 100,000 times per day to sustain life, the way we recognize a voice over the phone, and how the body coordinates itself to play music—all these topics and so many more can help a child of any age grow in appreciation for God's gift. Anything that a child, adolescent, or teenager enjoys as a part of everyday life—participating in or watching a sporting event, repairing something, playing a video game—can provide an opportunity to prompt them to thank God occasionally. In fact, one of the blessings of nighttime prayer with children is the opportunity to briefly mention all the good things that God has given us, none of which would be possible without the physical body.

2. *You know that your body is a sanctuary of the Holy Spirit who is in you, whom you have received from God, don't you? You do not*

belong to yourselves, For you have been bought with a price: there-
fore glorify God in your body (Corinthians 6:19-20).

Of all the body-related commentary in Scripture, these verses
from Saint Paul have probably been the most repeated. They are
frequently used by Christians who are into personal fitness as well
as by instructors who want to inspire their clients to be more active. However, there is much more for us in this passage than physical motivation. The context, the previous verses in this chapter six,
reveal Saint Paul's real point. First, the chapter is titled, "Sexual
Immorality." His entire message centers on his concern about inappropriate sexual relations (i.e., those outside of marriage) in the
communities around him. His general point, however, is that the
Christian's body is a temple, a sacred place in which God deigns to
come and live. Disrespectful physical acts can offend God the Holy
Spirit since the he dwells is within the body. However, it is not a
stretch to assume that Saint Paul intends that all aspects of a
healthy regard for the body (including sexual as well as physical
acts) should be elevated for the Christian.

For parents, two major teaching points can be drawn from this
part of Scripture. First, it provides an opportunity to discuss the
appropriate boundaries of physical contact within young relationships. A few years ago, a mom or two probably walked by their
teenager's room and heard John Mayer singing, "Your Body is a
Wonderland"? Try explaining those verses to an innocent, yet cu-
rious teen. Secondly, Saint Paul's words provide an ideal opportunity to engage in a conversation with teenagers, even young children, about the body as a gift. Simply expounding on the words

"glorify God in your body" can provide a powerful lesson to your child. Giving specific examples of how to glorify God with the body could include conversations about: 1) Why it's a good idea to follow a good nutrition program, 2) How a fitness regimen affects health in a positive way, 3) How good sleeping habits impact energy levels, 4) Why proper hygiene is necessary, 5) Why avoiding drugs and alcohol is just ... well, a *really* good idea, and so very many more things.

You simply cannot overemphasize the importance of mentioning the terms "God" and "body" in the same sentence to children. That is, it's not common in secular society to associate the two. Repetition serves as a gentle reminder that God is indeed alive and very present in our lives and that we should view our body as a blessing. It surely pleases him every time we acknowledge the human body as his most wonderful creation. Doing so simply and often (e.g., in regular brief prayers of thanksgiving) is so important.

3. *Christ has no body now on earth but yours, no hands but yours, no feet but yours, yours are the eyes through which Christ's compassion is to look out to the earth, yours are the feet by which He is to go about doing good and yours are the hands by which He is to bless us now.* Saint Teresa of Ávila

We recently found out that a young mother of five in a nearby parish had contracted a rare disease that caused poor circulation in her hands and feet. Tragically, both hands and one foot had to be amputated. The community, especially Catholic and other nearby churches, rallied to make her family meals for several months as well as raise money to assist with her medical expenses. We all know of similar situations where communities, nations, and even the entire world have been moved to help people in need. Each and every situation where someone's needs are being met is a living illustration of the above quote of Saint Teresa (1515-1582). In the New Testament, Christ, Saint Paul, and others insist that such actions are an integral part of being a follower of our Lord. Saint Teresa's words—for which she would surely credit the inspiration of the Holy Spirit— have so beautifully captured the essence of this truth that they have resonated in Christians for over four hundred years.

Theologically speaking, Saint Teresa is correct to assert that God (being pure spirit) relies on us to do his work on earth. Saying that "God has no hands but ours" does not only apply to our responsibility to mercifully respond to family crises or in the aftermath of natural disasters such as tsunamis and earthquakes. It happens a million times per day. Look around you. A nurse cares for a sick patient, someone assists in a local food drive for the poor, one neighbor helps another on moving day, or we make a meal for an elderly neighbor—these are the stories that *don't* make the news. God's fortunes are far greater than his perceived failings, but let's face it: bad news sells. Movies would not be movies if not for the violence and conflict that move the plot along frame by frames. It's boring to see people being nice to one another. So, like our cars and our bodies, we tend to take notice only when they are behaving poorly. That's right, it gets our attention when things are at their worst. Wouldn't you agree that it would be nice to promote and offer thanks (and NOT just on Thanksgiving) for all the *good* we are and that we can do?

Now more than ever parents have a host of volunteer opportunities to extend to their children. There are thousands of national organizations, churches, and Christian schools that organize and offer opportunities for young people to volunteer their services. Many Catholic High Schools, for example, now require some type of volunteering from every student. Moreover, national programs such as TeenLife, ISV, and Projects Abroad offer daily opportunities to meet these school requirements while enriching our children's experience. In addition, they also offer richer and more compelling experiences like longer summer programs in foreign lands. These opportunities raise awareness in our youth. They escalate gratitude even as they give an appreciation of how many people in this world are in desperate need. The central goal of this book is to improve the appreciation of the body and come to love what the body can do. A few hours or even several days of lending a helping hand can do much to calm poor body issues and re-focus young people on God's overall plan. Just as repeatedly viewing certain images can stir negative feelings about our body, frequent volunteering can move our mind to more mature pursuits and develop our soul for the better. So, it is worthwhile to become familiar with the local and national volunteer agencies. I encourage you to consider random one-day outings and long-term opportunities as a healthy part of your family dynamic.

4. Be who you are and be that well. St Francis de Sales

I have had several male and female friends who have more-or-less lived at the gym. After some time and hard work, their bodies looked great. But their circle of friends dwindled to their workout partners, who were only sometimes genuine friends. They spent more hours working out than anything else but work or school, and became so singularly obsessive about looking good that, frankly, they became boring. In conversation, they talked about their training. At dinner, they fretted over the slightest amount of salt or sugar. At social engagements, they spent more time looking into mirrors than into the eyes and conversations of other people. I began to notice a narcissistic quality that became less and less attractive, even as they became more outwardly attractive people. In time, I found myself gravitating away from them and growing closer to people who were more earthy, well-rounded, and real. I mean, how often have you seen a muscle-bound, perfectly chiseled person working in a soup line? Well, perhaps that's not fair, but a point is made. When self-absorption sets in, we can forget (or simply cease to care about) the importance of serving others.

Now, this is not to say that I don't encourage healthy exercise habits since sidestepping that would be to go against the basic tenets of my profession. It's just that now, more than ever, everything to do with our physical nature seems to be taken to the extreme. Tattoos (the size and number), muscularity, thinness, near-shocking eye color via special contact lenses, breast size, and the dozens of ways we attempt to defy aging and improve aesthetics are just a few that readily come to mind. Most troubling is that the inordinate amount of effort that goes into these extreme ventures often causes a shift in the way we see and serve God. Every act and each minute of anxiety tied to perfecting the body turns our attention away from and hardens our hearts to the things of God. Conversely, deeds of service and prayer for others turn our thoughts and hearts toward him. A turn toward and focus upon God is always healing to the soul and leads us further down the path of self-acceptance. When we know our actions are pleasing to God, we are more pleased with ourselves.

Now, way on the other side of the spectrum are the good souls that serve God but forget to serve themselves. In a soup line, we may see a kind gentleman who is dangerously overweight, unclean, and ladling soup with a cigarette dangling from his mouth. Is he serving God by serving others? Yes, quite literally. But even as he does so, he is abusing the body and ignoring the gift it is. It does no good in the long-run to rationalize the good deeds as a trade-off.

Our minds are an interesting place to be sometimes.

Parents who are balanced, keep things in perspective, and take care of their bodies while not obsessing over them usually pass these traits on to their children. Although we are aware that children go through phases of being influenced by their parents, we can never really know the effect we have on our kids. But as Saint Paul urges, we must always "fight the good fight of faith" (1 Tim 6:12) with the concentration, discipline, and extreme effort necessary to win the battle for the well-being of our children. As we do this—loving, teaching, disciplining, and modeling healthy habits for our children—we demonstrate the kind of love and acceptance that God has for his people.

Parents of children with disabilities have a particularly tough challenge. In an understatement for sure, navigating the world of disabilities obliges a parent to go well beyond what is required of other parents to instill a positive body image in their children. Although this book is about body image and *not* about disabilities, I would consider it negligent to not address the disabled, diseased, and disfigured in our discussion of body image.

One of the most memorable photos of Pope Francis's pontificate was one in which he kissed a grotesquely disfigured man who visited him at the Vatican. That man, Vinicio Riva, has a genetic disorder called neurofibromatosis Type 1 (or NF1). The pope, clearly acting spontaneously and with overwhelming compassion, probably made his encounter with Mr. Riva the signature event of his papacy.

The pope's actions were emotional and moving as he reached out to demonstrate the love that God wants to show one another. There were no expectations, no physical requirements, and no pretenses inherent in Pope Francis's actions. He simply embraced and showed love to a man that, like anyone else, deserves to be treated with dignity simply because he is a child of God. A moment like that puts the fixation on physical perfection firmly in its place, doesn't it? It can also help parents give perspective to their children when they complain about minor flaws on their face and body. Occasionally pointing out that millions of people deal with lost limbs, birth defects, and major scars from accidents or war can give our children a more well-rounded appreciation for their body as well as a compassion for others. You may even consider showing them a picture or a video of someone like Vinicio Riva to reinforce the lesson.

5. *We live in a society whose whole policy is to excite every nerve in the human body and keep it at the highest pitch of artificial tension, to strain every human desire to the limit and create as many new desires and synthetic passions as possible.* Thomas Merton, Trappist monk

Perhaps the most interesting point about Merton's comment is the era in which he said it. It was 1948, the year his famous book *The Seven Storey Mountain* was published. Most of us know the late 1940s through black and white photos. Many historians consider them to have been some of the most boring years of the 20th century. All this to say, the late 1940s don't seem like the kind of time that would inspire a monk to describe his surroundings as if he were currently living in New York City's Times Square. But it's possible that anyone with a pen and an audience could write something similar every decade since magazines with color photographs and motion pictures have been available. In many ways this comment by Merton reflects the theme of chapter four where I explain the many possible causes of a poor body image. At every turn in life, it seems someone or something is trying to stimulate our senses, neutralize God, and lead us away from all that is holy. When we overstimulate the body in an effort to look better, we end up emptying the soul.

The purpose of chapter four, and one of the central messages of this book for that matter, is to raise awareness of the fact that daily distractions are at work to convince us that our bodies are of little value unless they cause some type of arousal to those around us. Research has made it clear that exposing ourselves to particular images enlivens and encourages us in the wrong direction. These images of false perfection can have a substantial and unhealthy impact on the way we view others and ourselves.

Conscientious parents are constantly trying to monitor and balance their children's access to the internet, TV, movies, and certain magazines. That's because they are very aware that these media have the potential to excite every nerve in the bodies of their children. Any effort to limit availability to things that harm their developing body image can only be a step in the right direction. We are expected to protect our children and each year that we shelter them from damaging images limits their anxiety and protects their soul. And I urge you not to feel uncomfortable about raising clueless children—a common worry for conscientious parents. Our kids live in this world and, almost by osmosis, they pick up an awareness of their surroundings. It's almost helpful that they are aware of at least *some* negative images so that they can know what to stay away from.

Passion, about so many things is part of the human experience. Merton refers to "synthetic passions" which are what we need to be watchful of since passion has an uncanny ability to steer our thoughts and bodies away from God. As Saint Peter tells us, "Be of sober spirit, be on the alert. Your adversary, the devil, prowls around like a roaring lion, seeking someone to devour" (1 Pet 5:8).

For girls, the "devil" is the combination of images and the competition among other girls that develops in adolescence. She, unfortunately, learns a basic form of seduction way too early. For boys, the "devil" shows up in the pressure to use anabolic steroids and other performance enhancement products, pornography, and to attain to the perfection of Hollywood's shirtless hunk. He reaches and tempts girls through fashion magazines, select reality shows, and peer comparisons. Believing what the media tells us about how our body should look and be used is indeed a roaring lion. And it will devour our kids if we don't help them seek what God has to say about it.

6. *Athletic activity, in fact, highlights not only man's valuable physical abilities, but also his intellectual and spiritual capacities. It is not just physical strength and muscular efficiency, but it also has a soul and must show its complete face. This is why a true athlete must not let himself be carried away by an obsession with physical perfection, or be enslaved by the rigid laws of production and consumption, or by purely utilitarian and hedonistic considerations.* Saint John Paul II, to a group of athletes in 2000

Pope Saint John Paul II has left a legacy of great writings (e.g., *Theology of the Body*) and encyclicals (e.g., *The Splendor of Truth*). He has traveled more than any other pontiff and canonized more saints than all of his predecessors over the last 900 years combined. And, as many know, he had a genuine passion for sports and being physically active. In fact, in 2004, during the final full-year of Saint

John Paul II's papacy, The Office of Church and Sport was instituted in response to the highly influential nature of exercise and sport on contemporary culture. One of the primary responsibilities of this office is to "foster a sports culture, as a means of bringing about the holistic growth of the person."[1] Simply put, the Catholic Church has extended its teaching of basic ethics and morals to the realm of sport and exercise. Saint John Paul II's comment above says that athletic competition "must show its complete face." This means that sports and Christian living are not mutually exclusive but must be integrated and conjoined willingly by each participant.

Further, the Office of Church and Sport's message is meant not just for competitive athletes, but also for those whose athleticism is limited to exercise. In both arenas, we have seen the use of testosterone/anabolic steroids and human growth hormone (HGH) as a means to enhance performance. It is common for people to argue that having access to a superior nutritional plan, better training facilities, and more experienced strength and conditioning personnel are themselves performance enhancers.

While each of these things lends their own set of advantages to the athlete, none is illegal nor should they be. It's natural and noble to improve ability through hard work, good eating, and seeking the wisdom of good trainers. On the other hand, there is reason why the NHL, NBA, NFL, MLB, and International Olympic Committee have banned the aforementioned drugs. That is because they are

---

[1] The Pontifical Council for the Laity: The Office of Church and Sport. See http://www.laici.va/content/laici/en/sezioni/chiesa-e-sport.html.

known to cause harm to the body and not because of their proven ability to improve performance.

Interestingly, there are several readily available products that have been clearly established as ergogenic aids yet are not banned by any organization since their use causes little or no side effects. Creatine monohydrate (a common and well-known compound shown to improve ability) and sodium bicarbonate (baking soda, also known to assist athletes in brief, high intensity bouts of activity) are two of them. While the real motive of professional sports organizations in banning steroids and HGH may have more to do with legality than the physical protection of their athletes, their action is still appropriate, necessary, and honorable.

Perhaps the most poignant words in Saint John Paul II's quote are a warning against being *"enslaved by the rigid laws of production and consumption, or by purely utilitarian and hedonistic considerations."* That is, the Catholic Church views competition not as an act by which we nurture some selfish cause (e.g. making money) or serve our egos (e.g. becoming famous). Instead, we are to use our bodies in one of the many ways that glorify God.

Participation in sports and physical exercise should be considered a blessing, a way to improve our health, and a means to experience competition while fostering relationships among the participants. Most Christian athletes and coaches would readily agree with this philosophy, but few have articulated the purpose and meaning of the body in the context of sport and exercise as well as the Catholic Church.

Parents want their sons and daughters to win in sport and to have their bodies respond to training as much as anyone. But it's the win-at-all-costs mentality that is contrary to the teachings of the Catholic Church and does injustice to the basic principles of competition. From the time they first begin to compete, we should be having strategic conversations with our children that teach them that winning does not mean you are a winner and losing does not mean you are a loser. Granted, this can be a tough sell to a little leaguer who just lost the district championship. But painting the overall goals of competition for your children on a regular basis will do them a great service now and in the future. After all, bad losers in little league and other youth sports often grow up to be bad losers as adults in key professions such as teaching, politics, business managers, coaches, and so on. One simple way to make the world a better place to live is to raise children who know how to be good winners *and* good losers.

Finally, the win-at-all-costs principle extends to the misuse of steroids and HGH, which are used to either improve performance and/or to look better—even though they are illegal, can be harmful, and are considered immoral by many. Whatever the reason for their use, it's well worth your time to educate your child on their side effects. It is also important to point out that their use goes against the basic convictions of what it means to be a good competitor. The ole "give it your best and that's enough for me" is dated for sure. But like a lot of old sayings, this one still has merit, and it is spot on.

7. Moral concerns arise due to the risk of addiction which threatens authentic freedom and constitutes a serious form of human bondage.
Father Tadeusz Pacholczyk, PhD in Neuroscience

I once read that we are *all* addicted to something. After reading this, I remember thinking "What a ridiculous comment." But after giving it more thought, I recognized the truth in this statement. Addictions go well beyond drugs, alcohol, pornography, and food. Just think, for a moment, about a little-known affliction called "Runners' Addiction." Running, you might say, is a good endeavor. It clears the lungs, stimulates blood flow, keeps the weight down, and makes us feel good through the release of endorphins. I know because I jog on a regular basis. Yet, there are some people who have jogged *every day* for the past thirty years (see "United States Running Streak Association" online). Think about it; if it's every day, haven't they run on important holidays, birthdays, and anniversaries and despite illness? And like so many other addictions, wouldn't that kind of single-mindedness run the risk of affecting their marriages, friends, work, and other relationships? And, is that kind of dedication to a sport sending the right kind of message to their children? When anything—good or bad—becomes the most important thing in your life, you may be facing an addiction.

Furthermore, plenty of people become addicted to perfecting their faces as well. And it's not just in the form of thousands of dollars spent on anti-aging cream, hair transplants, and anabolic steroids. Some lost souls actually allow surgeons to cut them open in an effort to improve their looks. How insane is that? Inordinate and anxious thoughts about our body image can morph into addiction as well. I've attempted to paint vivid pictures of the levels of stress and discontent that body distortion causes many people, but the quote by Father Pacholczyk crystallizes it: addiction *"threatens authentic freedom and constitutes a serious form of bondage."* To clarify this point, look at what the Catholic Catechism says about freedom:

"As long as freedom has not bound itself definitively to its ultimate good which is God, there is the possibility of *choosing between good and evil*, and thus of growing in perfection or of failing and sinning. This freedom characterizes properly human acts."[2]

And . . .

"The more one does what is good, the freer one becomes. There is no true freedom except in the service of what is good and just."[3]

As practicing Christians, we are in a constant battle to do what is right. But living a life of virtue goes beyond the efforts to avoid lying, stealing, and cheating. It also ventures into areas such as negative body image. Struggling with body distortion can manifest itself in numerous ways, from persistent thoughts to regular, even daily attempts to perfect the body. And all these obsessive thoughts and consequent actions bind us to the unworthy and take us further away from choosing God's desire for us. This is exactly where freedom comes in. Chasing the impossible (in this case, the perfect body) stifles or even halts our minds and souls from seeking God and his daily message to us. This is why all efforts by parents to

---

[2] Catechism of the Catholic Church, No. 1732.
[3] Catechism of the Catholic Church, No. 1733.

teach their children such principles as authentic freedom, choosing the good, and the results of sin, are worth their time and energy.

Friends of mine, Steve and Andrea, who are parents of three children, are concerned about their youngest daughter Meaghan. Meaghan suffers from a poor body image despite being raised in a home with loving, accepting parents. She has had relatively limited access to the media and was well-catechized in the Faith. If nothing else, this shows the relentless negative impact today's culture exerts on the body image of our young people. It also shows their frailty and susceptibility. Steven and Andrea can still see the effect that this issue has on Meaghan who is now in her thirties. They have witnessed a happy and carefree little girl tragically morph into a young woman who is trapped in the world of body image distortion. She is a casualty in human bondage. Like so many parents, Steve and Andrea fully realize that teachable moments are fleeting. And they are very aware that even the best parents don't always know what to do—even when the problem is well-defined and standing right in front of them. As an older parent of young children, I might be more apt to feel empowered by experience and virtue; I might be tempted to believe that combination will help me always do the right thing at the right time. But, in reality, I still feel lost and clueless in some situations. I've learned that coming up with the right solution at the right time is a real and ongoing challenge for parents. But I've also learned that parenting principles and practices centered on God, his word, and his healing power are powerful tools. God longs to see an intense desire in us to seek the good and he will meet us there with the help we need. Bringing all our parenting challenges to him makes breaking the cycle of anxiety a little easier and will create a more peaceful household.

In the case of Steve and Andrea, I don't know all the specifics of Meaghan's body image concerns, and they didn't ask for my help; they simply shared their story. However, it was clear to see that they were very confused by their daughter, and it pained them to talk about it all. While Meaghan has not been paralyzed by her body image issues—in fact, she is a pleasant, productive young woman—her struggle has affected her life enough that her parents have taken notice and, unfortunately, accepted some of the blame. Sometimes, like in the instance of Meaghan, no one or everyone is to blame. But Steve and Andrea can take comfort in the fact that they are good, loving parents, deeply faithful to the Catholic Church, and devotedly taught that faith to their children. Yes, like all of us, they would probably like a do-over on a few occasions, but they have managed to raise wonderful children. Perhaps the moral here is for all parents in similar circumstances to embrace the imperfections inherent in parenting. Take solace that you have taught and practiced the Catholic faith and rely on God's healing power to close the gap in his time.

8. The beginning of love is to let those we love be perfectly themselves, and not to twist them to fit our own image. Otherwise, we love only the reflection of ourselves we find in them. Thomas Merton, Trappist monk

Of the quotes in this chapter, no single one speaks more directly to our role as a parent than this. The irony here is that few parents consider that they may be the source of their child's body image problem. It's sometimes easier to blame the media, peer comparisons, and the prevalence of plastic surgery and anabolic steroids. Still, parents can (sometimes unwittingly) say things that have a profound and lasting impact on their children. A young woman who has struggled with maintaining an "ideal" weight most of her adult life once talked about such a comment. She said that despite all the looks and comments she has received, the one she most vividly recalls came from her father when she was a teen. He told her that being overweight was a sign that she lacked control and that it made a statement to society that she was careless and lazy. While it could be argued that there is some truth in these statements, the reason her father's comments had such an impact is that it was clear that *her father* was the one who felt that way, not society. In these careless words to his daughter, he revealed that he neither respected women nor found them attractive if they were overweight. This form of projection can have a profound effect on any young person—especially a teenager who is looking for love and acceptance from the most important people in her life, her parents.

Much of what I'd like to say related to this quote, I've already said elsewhere. But it does bear repeating that our worth and dignity are not tied to our youthful appearance or physical attractiveness. Remember the overweight, unshaven, cigarette-smoking soup line volunteer? He may not be the picture of health, but his good deeds still hold value. One of the many ways that parents can reflect the same love that God has for us is to love their children unconditionally while still guiding them toward maturity. Proper eating habits, regular physical activity, and avoiding drugs and excess alcohol are healthy behaviors that should be modeled, taught, and encouraged.

9. *The body, in fact, and it alone, is capable of making visible what is invisible: the spiritual and the divine. [The body] was created to transfer in the visible reality of the world the invisible mystery hidden since time immemorial in God, and thus be a sign of it.* Saint Pope John Paul II (General Audience 2/20/80)

These words, spoken to a General Audience in Rome in 1980, are always used as part of Saint John Paul II's *Theology of the Body*. In fact, this particular quote is one of the many that have become the core message of *Theology of the Body* books and related materials. It's here that JPII points out that we cannot see spiritual things with our eyes. A spiritual being such as God is by nature invisible. But since the body is visible it is key mode in which God reveals himself to us. And through us.

There's an old saying, "The eyes are the window to the soul." But in truth, the whole body is the window to the soul. How we think and, thus, what we say and what we do are direct reflections of who we really are. Specifically, the physical body reveals the spiritual nature of the person. As body-persons we are made in the image of the invisible God, and as TOB scholar Christopher West puts it, "This striking declaration brings us to the summit of John Paul's anthropology (his understanding of man), crystallizing everything he has to say about the body. The human body reveals the mystery of God!"[4]

The Scriptures reveal that the creation of the human body is a direct act of God. In effect, this is the initial "good news" from our Lord. Not only does God love us enough to send us his only Son in bodily form, but he also gave us a body so that we could fully comprehend the concept of a savior. As with our savior, our body is a physical means to embrace life through all that we experience as human beings. In short, we should use, not abuse, such a wonderful gift.

Some of this language may be a bit beyond the ability of children to fully comprehend, but they are certainly capable of grasping the main theological point. The body is the greatest gift we receive from God; therefore, we show our gratitude and honor this gift by living out a virtuous life (e.g., extending forgiveness, charity, and kindness to others). Without the guidance and encouragement of parents to make a life of virtue a real thing, children often live out of their sinful nature and embrace envy, pride, and greed. Such inner motivations lead to outward behaviors because the body follows what's in the soul. And one way this plays out is when they become preoccupied with perfecting the body rather than simply taking care of it.

10. *Therefore I urge you, brethren, by the mercies of God, to present your bodies a living and holy sacrifice, acceptable to God, which is*

---

[4] West, C. (2001). The Pope's Theology of the Body. Retrieved from http://catholiceducation.org/articles/sexuality/se0058.html

your spiritual service of worship. Do not be conformed to this world, but continuously be transformed by the renewing of your minds so that you may be able to determine what God's will is—what is proper, pleasing, and perfect. Romans 12:1-2

It's rather easy to say that we should not be "conformed to this world," isn't it? But with further thought, few quotes are more challenging than this one. While I'm at it, why don't I throw in "Give away all of your possessions and follow me" (Matt 19:21)? But returning to the original quote, we are all very much a part of this world and its values and we constantly feel the pressure of being squeezed into its mold. I think it's a fair assumption that all readers of this book live in an industrialized society, which means there are far more distractions to our souls than ever. The Gospels and a sacramental life, in turn, are the remedy. Christ and each writer of the New Testament teaches us how to exercise our faith in a variety of situations, and virtually all of them are relevant to today's experiences. This is the beauty of Scripture, and *this* is the Good News. The written word of God gives us Christ's commands, and the Holy Spirit through the sacraments gives us the ability to understand them and the power to live them out in this world. This combination is compelling and a defining mark of the Catholic faith. Further, to "...continuously be transformed by the renewing of your minds" could be understood as encouragement to not just participate in the sacraments like reconciliation and the Eucharist, but to do so wholeheartedly and often—even daily if possible. As for those who are given the responsibility to raise children, consider this from the Catholic Catechism:

The fecundity of conjugal love cannot be reduced solely to the procreation of children, but must extend to their moral education and their spiritual formation. "The role of parents in education is of such importance that it is almost impossible to provide an adequate substitute.[5] *The right and the duty of parents to educate their children are primordial and inalienable.*[6]

As every parent knows, continually guiding the words and actions of a child is a daunting but necessary task. However, when times get tough and complex (hint: the time in life when pop boy bands like One Direction and BTS are relevant), some parents start giving in, or stop trying at all. God's will—doing what is "proper, pleasing, and perfect"—is a tough concept to fully understand and even tougher to live out. But doing this instead of being conformed to the world's thinking and values is the direct command of God. And just one way we work this out in life is to stay clear of what society says is the purpose of the body. From the time your children are young, you will have to exert continual attention and effort to help them develop a positive body image. Even so, there are no guarantees that this or any other worthy task in life will be easy. But take heart—you and your child are assured that you will not go at it alone (Ps 34:17-19; Matt 11:28).

Don't let the media or anything else determine your worth. Let God do that.

---

[5] *Gravissimum Educationis* (1965). *Second Vatican Council's Declaration on Christian Education.*

[6] *Catechism of the Catholic Church*, No. 2222.

Chapter 10

You Can't Have it All

You also, as living stones, are being built up as a spiritual house
for a holy priesthood, to offer up spiritual sacrifices
acceptable to God through Jesus Christ.

1 Peter 2:5

I was recently invited to give a presentation to a youth group about body image. My goal was to get them to grapple with all the gifts of the human body. So, I asked them to come up with one sport, hobby, or pastime that they most enjoy. One by one, I asked many of the thirty-five to forty young people present to call out their response to the question. There were many repeats (e.g., soccer and computer games), but there were also some unique responses such as computer programming, oil painting, and building model planes.

Following their responses, I expounded on what was obvious. The human body—with all its responsiveness, versatility, and ability to improve in skill—should be appreciated. We all have so much to be thankful for that directly involves the senses, a muscle group, or the marvelous brain. In addition, I also reminded them that the body is capable of healing itself, helping others, and enjoying our favorite foods. With that, they smiled (I think mainly at the food comment). But I really feel they "got it." And so can you and so can your child. Continually teaching the concept of body-as-a-gift is well worth your time and energy. If our children have an inadequate view of or appreciation for their bodies, we parents have the opportunity and responsibility to correct their wrong thinking.

When to get help

So, how do we gauge the severity of a poor body image in children? Body Dysmorphic Disorder was officially recognized as a psychological issue in 1997 and continues to lag behind in research, the number of professionals that have committed to its cause, and even a comprehensive understanding. This is all the more significant when we consider its effect on the most vulnerable members of our society. Because managing poor body image issues on their own may not be possible for some, here are some clues that may indicate whether the problem goes beyond the suggestions of this book. Children may have body dysmorphic disorder if they:

- ➢ Constantly compare their appearance with others
- ➢ Refuse to let their picture be taken, or are extremely self-conscious in photos
- ➢ Keep checking or discussing a certain body part that they think is flawed
- ➢ Make drastic attempts to hide the perceived flaws
- ➢ Feel anxious and self-conscious around other people
- ➢ Avoid or limit leaving the house unless it's necessary since body dysmorphic disorder has been known to limit social interaction and romantic relationships

> ➢ Refer to themselves as "hideous," "ugly," "disgusting," or with other negative terms
> ➢ Seek or hint at the need for cosmetic surgery to look perfect: liposuction, rhinoplasty, etc.

If you observe one or more of the above behaviors in your child, some professionals feel that a degree of body disorder likely exists, and some form of psychological treatment should be considered. While some may require a more aggressive form of therapy to combat this issue, I am not suggesting that you make any definitive decisions based on the questions or information provided here. Still, let's investigate this further by considering the following questions:

Has your child admitted, in some fashion, that they struggle with body dysmorphic disorder? This is where the saying, "The truth can set you free" comes in. Simply put, healing body image problems starts with honesty and acceptance. This is a great first step.

Will talking about this to trusted family members help? Children often need sounding boards and want to feel that they are not alone in the issues they grapple with. Explaining to your child how you feel about your body is a step toward healing. Feelings of imperfection are common. Comments from other kids and media-related images will make them feel inadequate. Planting this seed often and early opens the door to healthy conversations. God's love, expressed through a parent and other loved ones, plays an important part in healing body image problems.

Does your child treat himself or herself well? Committing to a healthy lifestyle such as eating well and exercising regularly can calm many of the anxieties that accompany a poor body image.

Can your child identify the main culprits that have led to the formation of a poor body image? For example, limiting or even purging from their life things that trigger obsessive negative thoughts about their body (e.g., participating in conversations about beauty/attractiveness, fashion/muscle magazines, physically appealing TV shows, etc.) can only help. And a follow-up question may be…

As a parent, can you commit to embracing the theme of *Theology of the Body* and Scripture as it addresses the body? The full intention of this book is to use the Word of God and Pope Saint John Paul II's *TOB* to transform our thoughts so that we see our body as a gift—regardless of our body fat percentage, level of attractiveness, height, and other bodily qualities.

Know that you're not in this alone

Turning to God when we need strength accomplishes two major goals for parents. First, we turn to the best source of wisdom and strength (Ps 37:39; Phil 4:13) especially when the task seems too big to conquer (Matt 19:26); and second, we demonstrate that faith to our children. Children learn many habits from their parents, so why should living out our Catholic faith be any different? I've witnessed several sets of parents struggle with their child's body distortion issues as if they were their own. Actually, that makes sense because our love for children leads us to experience their pain as if it were our own. The greatest gift we can give our children (and ourselves) is to live a life of constant and meaningful prayer and to regularly receive the sacraments and allow the grace that God promises us to take hold.

Every parent can gain from additional wisdom and fortitude. Pray for the wisdom you need to implement ways to temper TV-watching and decide which movies to allow. Pray also for discernment regarding whether Disney and other animated characters might play a role in your child's body image, and when and how to limit those images that seem to be having the most negative impact. Often, discussing these things with your spouse will bring a great deal of peace and insight as well. Remember, there is power in numbers. Lastly, fortitude will help you follow through on the insight wisdom has given you.

Get support when needed

Even though so many young people suffer from body distortion, it is not a common topic of discussion on talk shows, blogs, or in presentations to parish communities. Sadly, it remains a dark secret for many. You probably won't get much helpful support or information unless you directly seek it. There are several books available, many that directly address the issue of body image from both secular and Christian standpoints. There's no guaranteed way to create a positive body image—from the Catholic perspective or any other—and it is not my intention to make that claim in this book. But this and other efforts can provide insight and perhaps come to it from an angle that hits your household in the right way at the right time. From a Christian viewpoint, Consider *Weightless: Making Peace with Your Body* by Catholic author Kate Wicker, *Thinking Theologically About Body Image* by Michael Poteet, and *Wanting to be Her: Body Image Secrets Victoria Won't Tell You* by Michelle Graham. To further investigate TOB for youth, there's *Theology of the Body for Teens: Middle School Edition* and *Theology of the Body for Teens: High School Edition* both by Catholic writers Brian Butler, Jason Evert, and Christina Evert. From a secular (and more academic) stance, check out *Understanding Body Dissatisfaction in Men, Women and Children* by Sarah Grogan, and *The Adonis Complex: The Secret Crisis of Male Body Obsession* by Harrison Pope, Katharine Phillips, and Roberto Olivardia. (Note: Although *The Adonis Complex* has been in print for over two decades, students in my body image class consistently say it's the most interesting reading in the course. And I agree; it is a worthwhile read).

Know that your efforts will count for something

Having four children and teaching for twenty years has made me realize that parenting and teaching have a few similarities. As a professor, I have often been taken a little off guard when former students share—whether just after a semester concludes or years later—that they were touched, motivated, or simply educated in a special way by the content of a class. It's especially surprising when my recollection of those same students is that they seemed disinterested in the class, and sometimes appeared to disdain it. Every parent knows that some actions they take (read: discipline) will not be fully understood and rarely appreciated by their children. But even a little bit of parental insight tells us that such actions are necessary to raise moral and ethical children.

This premise extends to creating a positive body image. Just suggest that a specific television program, movie, or attire is inappropriate, and you'll likely be met with a resistance that would make a world power in battle take notice! But comfort yourself with the fact that you're protecting their soul and that efforts early in their lives are necessary and most effective (Prov 19:18, 22:6). You've surely noted that this book contains as many "dos" (suggestions for improving body image) as "don'ts" (things to avoid to keep a poor body image from developing). One of the more interesting aspects of developing a healthy body image is that the goal is often to limit something rather than to progress in something. For this reason, parents may never really know how their efforts have paid off. How can we gauge how much impact *omitting* something has? That's parenting though, isn't it? While we can't protect our children from everything that would harm their souls, we can persevere in focused instruction about what is bad as well as what is good and make concerted efforts to model and teach the difference.

You can't have it all...but you can have what's important

We're not perfect—in body or soul—and neither are our children. No magical solution exists for improving body image. I wish I could offer one; but I can't, and neither can anyone else. But I do wholeheartedly believe that it's manageable through a combination of omitting some harmful things and inserting other healthy things. Above all, never relent on establishing a family that is sustained on a vital relationship with God. Ignore (and even abhor) any hint of the "You Can Have It All" philosophy. If you're make yourself a slave to exercise and extreme dieting, you will have little time or interest in God and other things of value like friendships, family life, or even a worthy hobby. Yes, you may attain a near perfect body as the result of daily, focused workouts and nutrition—but there will always be a price to pay. Often, it's a big one. A person marked by moderation in all things is generally a healthy person. Period.

I once saw an article in a popular women's magazine titled, "How to Love the Skin You're In." I read the article and was fairly impressed overall. The article hit the target by using terms like "acceptance," "everyone's different," and "perfection is not possible." But other than missing some depth, it omitted a vital component: God. You can talk about the body and all its wonderful capabilities. You can even express great appreciation for it. But if you fail to include language that recognizes the body as a gift from God and his greatest creation, your conversation will fall short of meaningful.

The irony is that most of the readers of that particular article (this is a projection here) would likely welcome God into the discussion. They would even be apt to agree that for true healing to occur, God must be included. In fact, I am sure that we would all agree that a truly healthy person is not just physically healthy, but also spiritually healthy. We simply must include God in discussions of complex issues like body image. That's the purpose of this book, and that's why you've read it.

Does this book provide all the answers? I am sure it doesn't. But I've tried my best to base most of my suggestions and solutions on God, teachings of the Catholic Church, Scripture, and the Sacraments—something not attempted before.

And now for a little summary:

Keep in mind that there are too many factors that we, as parents, cannot control completely—media images, conversations with ill-intentioned people, messages from social media, and steroid use by athletes and models. But we *can* control many things within our own families—time spent in prayer and adoration, Mass attendance, volunteer outings, individual and family physical activity sessions, and strategic TV and internet time. We can avoid the things that trigger a poor body image and spend quality time with God, family, and friends. When we do, our attention is channeled in a positive way. And we are more likely to shift our priorities away from selfish pursuits of perfection and toward the needs of others.

You can't have it all—but you *can* have what's important.

And a final comment:

I appreciate the fact that you've sought this book. It means that you care a great deal about your child and that you are acutely aware of God's role in your child's life. Every parent who reads or even desires to read this book inspires me. God bless you in your journey to raise healthy children—not just on the issue of body image, but in all things.

www.ingramcontent.com/pod-product-compliance
Lightning Source LLC
Chambersburg PA
CBHW071235290326
41931CB00038B/3036